Practice questions in Psychopharmacology

Volume 2

Dr. Srikanth Sajja
Humber NHS Foundation Trust
Hull, UK

Professor Ann M Mortimer
Foundation Chair
Head of the Department of Psychiatry
University of Hull
Hull, UK

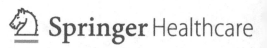
Springer Healthcare

Published by Springer Healthcare Ltd, 236 Gray's Inn Road, London, WC1X 8HB, UK.

www.springerhealthcare.com

© 2011 Springer Healthcare, a part of Springer Science+Business Media.

British Library Cataloguing-in-Publication Data.

A catalogue record for this book is available from the British Library.

Cover photo by Srikanth Sajja LRPS.

Project editor: Hannah Cole
Designer: Joe Harvey
Artworker: Sissan Mollerfors
Production: Marina Maher

Foreword

This book is a welcome addition to currently available resources in psychopharmacology for trainees. Questions on psychopharmacology (including basic and clinical psychopharmacology and therapeutics) are common topics in the psychiatry field and many trainees have difficulties with them.

Dr Sajja is to be commended for producing an excellent series of relevant questions and has used an extensive bibliography to generate topics that will be both a useful test of progression as well as a memory aid and primer.

I often think the best answer to any psychopharmacology question is "I'll look it up!" Given the size of the Data Sheet Compendium and other psychopharmacology volumes, this is a sensible strategy for clinical management. However, this is not a recourse that one can use in an exam, although this book should help considerably with most major examinations in this field.

Professor I. Nicol Ferrier
Academic Psychiatry, Institute of Neuroscience
Newcastle General Hospital
Newcastle, UK

Acknowledgements

I would very much like to thank Professor Ann Mortimer for making valuable suggestions and being a source of inspiration by joining me as a co-author.

I am grateful to the post-graduate trainees, my colleagues and leading academicians in psychopharmacology for their useful feedback and encouragement.

I also thank Dr Dave Armstrong for his assistance in preparing some questions related to alcohol and drug abuse.

I am deeply indebted to Professor Nicol Ferrier for kindly providing the Foreword to the book.

I gratefully acknowledge the encouragement received from my parents and the patience shown by my wife and my daughter during the completion of this task.

I also thank my secretary Sheila Jenkinson for preparing this manuscript in time.

My special thanks to Hannah Cole, my publisher, for her guidance and support.

And finally, I owe my gratitude to my patients for making me constantly think and update my knowledge in this wonderful and challenging field of psychopharmacology.

Srikanth Sajja
2011

Preface

Psychopharmacology is a fascinating and exciting speciality that is constantly undergoing new and rapid scientific developments with clinical applications. The aim of this book is to provide practice questions in psychopharmacology to facilitate learning and revision. It consists of 2600 questions in the form of 'True/False Individual Statements, Extended Matching Items and Best of Five' formats, organised in 52 papers in two volumes.

Every attempt has been made to cover all relevant topics in psychopharmacology, addressing both knowledge and clinical competency related to the speciality. Resources used to prepare the questions are provided in the 'reading list' at the end, giving access to extensive cross-references.

This book will be a useful means of self-assessment for both trainees and practitioners in the fields of psychiatry, neurology, pharmacology, psychiatric pharmacy and general medicine.

Srikanth Sajja
2011

Topics covered

Development of Psychotropic Drugs

Research Methodology for Drug Trials

Receptors

Pharmacokinetics

Pharmacodynamics

Pharmacogenetics

Anxiolytics, hypnotics

Antipsychotic drugs

Mood Stabilisers

Antidepressant Drugs

Antimuscarinic Drugs

Antiepileptic Drugs

Drugs Used in Movement Disorders

Drugs Used in Substance Dependence

Antidementia Drugs

Adverse Reactions

Drug Interactions

Pharmacological Treatment of Psychiatric Disorders

Psychopharmacology of Children

Psychopharmocology of Elderly

Psychopharmacology of Women

Psychotropic Drugs in Special Patient Groups

New Drugs

Pharmacoeconomics

Psycho Socio Cultural Aspects of Psychopharmacology

Paper 27

	True	False

1. Lithium can raise serum calcium levels. ☐ ☐

2. Anticholinergic drugs have no effect on the akinesia in the treatment of Parkinson's disease. ☐ ☐

3. Norepinephrine transport pump is separate and distinct from tyrosine transport pump. ☐ ☐

4. Naloxone is a long-acting μ receptor antagonist. ☐ ☐

5. Tranylcypromine is contraindicated in patients with Parkinson's disease who are on L-dopa treatment. ☐ ☐

6. Antidepressant medication is effective in treatment of bulimia nervosa even in the absence of depressive symptoms. ☐ ☐

7. Amisulpiride shows selective antagonism of inhibitory dopamine (D_2) autoreceptors in the prefrontal cortex. ☐ ☐

8. Stimulant drugs used in the treatment for ADHD reduce hyperactive behaviour without influencing information processing. ☐ ☐

9. Acamprosate reduces the excitatory actions of glutamate at the NMDA receptor. ☐ ☐

10. Cholinergic nicotinic receptors are fast receptors unlike cholinergic muscarinic receptors which are slow receptors. ☐ ☐

11. Poor response to behaviour therapy predicts poor response to pharmacotherapy in treatment for obsessive-compulsive disorder. ☐ ☐

12. Antipsychotic effect of a neuroleptic takes longer than the time of onset of the antipsychotic induced prolactin rise. ☐ ☐

13. Severe depression is a recognized feature of propranolol toxicity. ☐ ☐

14. Clonidine reduces both REM latency and slow-wave sleep. ☐ ☐

15. Side effects of valproate include hair loss and weight gain. ☐ ☐

16. G-protein coupled receptors include both adrenergic and $5HT_2$ receptors. ☐ ☐

17. Zaleplon has longer elimination half-life than zolpidem and zopiclone. ☐ ☐

18. D_4 receptors bind clozapine with higher affinity than cloned D_2 receptors. ☐ ☐

19. The specific location of the serotonin transporter gene (SLC6A4) is on the short arm of chromosome 13. ☐ ☐

20. Cyproheptadine has been associated with weight loss. ☐ ☐

21. Leptin is a peptide that belongs to the interleukin 6 cytokine family. ☐ ☐

22. Glycine is an excitatory transmitter in spinal cord. ☐ ☐

23. Acetazolamide is a carbonic anhydrase inhibitor licensed for use in conjunction with other antiepileptic drugs. ☐ ☐

24. Naltrexone is a long acting orally administered μ receptor antagonist. ☐ ☐

25. Dopamine auto receptor antagonists increase both REM and non-REM sleep. ☐ ☐

26. Opiate antagonists are associated with short-term reduction in binge eating. ☐ ☐

27. Alpha2 adrenoceptor antagonists have shown efficacy in improving memory in schizophrenic patients. ☐ ☐

28. Receptors are protein molecules synthesized in the cell body of the neuron. ☐ ☐

29. Nausea and vomiting are major side effects of ergolines (bromocriptine, lisuride and pergolide). ☐ ☐

30. Desmopressin has shown efficacy in reducing the frequency of the enuresis at night. ☐ ☐

31. Concurrent administration of lithium with an SSRI can result in serotonin syndrome. ☐ ☐

32. Valproic acid increases slow wave sleep in adults but decreases it in children. ☐ ☐

33. Low Ki value of a drug reflects its greater affinity for the receptor. ☐ ☐

34. Stimulation of the κ receptors generates reinforcing properties. ☐ ☐

35. Rivastigmine is a pseudo-irreversible inhibitor of both acetyl and butyryl cholinesterases. ☐ ☐

36. Clonidine worsens the severity of tics in persons with tic disorder and comorbid ADHD. ☐ ☐

37. S-demethylcitalopram is the main metabolite of escitalopram. ☐ ☐

38. Symptoms of anticholinergic intoxication include mydriasis. ☐ ☐

39. Lithium reduces the functional activity of postsynaptic beta receptors. ☐ ☐

40. Mirtazapine acts as an antagonist of histamine H_1 receptors. ☐ ☐

41. MAOIs should be discontinued at least two weeks before starting carbamazepine treatment. ☐ ☐

42. Fluoxetine induces elevated mood in non-depressed healthy individuals. ☐ ☐

43. Drugs which lower serum amylase levels include valproate. ☐ ☐

44. Opioids are derivatives of the naturally occurring compound opium. ☐ ☐

45. Hypnotic drugs decrease stage 1 of non-REM sleep and prolong stage 2 sleep. ☐ ☐

46. Tolerance of the tuberoinfundibular dopaminergic system to the action of neuroleptics does not develop. ☐ ☐

47. The low incidence of side effects with SSRIs is due to their lack of antihistaminergic and anti – α_1 adrenergic receptor activities. ☐ ☐

48. Increased fat to lean body mass ratio is associated with decrease in the half-lives of lipophilic drugs. ☐ ☐

49. Flumazenil reverses the anticonvulsant effect of clonazepam. ☐ ☐

50. Venlafaxine is a bicyclic phenyl ethylamine derivative. ☐ ☐

Paper 27

1. Lithium can raise serum calcium levels.
Ans. **True.** By causing hyperparathyroidism.

2. Anticholinergic drugs have no effect on the akinesia in the treatment of Parkinson's disease.
Ans. **True.**

3. Norepinephrine transport pump is separate and distinct from tyrosine transport pump.
Ans. **True.**

4. Naloxone is a long-acting μ receptor antagonist.
Ans. **False.** It is short-acting (2 – 4 hours).

5. Tranylcypromine is contraindicated in patients with Parkinson's disease who are on L-dopa treatment.
Ans. **True.**

6. Antidepressant medication is effective in treatment of bulimia nervosa even in the absence of depressive symptoms.
Ans. **True.**

7. Amisulpiride shows selective antagonism of inhibitory dopamine (D_2) autoreceptors in the prefrontal cortex.
Ans. **True.** To reduce the negative symptoms.

8. Stimulant drugs used in the treatment for ADHD reduce hyperactive behaviour without influencing information processing.
Ans. **False.** Enhance information processing.

9. Acamprosate reduces the excitatory actions of glutamate at the NMDA receptor.
Ans. **True.**

10. Cholinergic nicotinic receptors are fast receptors unlike cholinergic muscarinic receptors which are slow receptors.
Ans. **True.**

11. Poor response to behaviour therapy predicts poor response to pharmacotherapy in treatment for obsessive-compulsive disorder.
Ans. **False.**

12. Antipsychotic effect of a neuroleptic takes longer than the time of onset of the antipsychotic induced prolactin rise.
Ans. **True.**

13. Severe depression is a recognized feature of propranolol toxicity.
Ans. **True.**

14. Clonidine reduces both REM latency and slow-wave sleep.
Ans. **False.** It increases these.

15. Side effects of valproate include hair loss and weight gain.
Ans. **True.**

16. G-protein coupled receptors include both adrenergic and $5HT_2$ receptors.
Ans. **True.**

17. Zaleplon has longer elimination half-life than zolpidem and zopiclone.
Ans. **False.** It has a shorter half-life of 1 hour.

18. D_4 receptors bind clozapine with higher affinity than cloned D_2 receptors.

Ans. True.

19. The specific location of the serotonin transporter gene (SLC6A4) is on the short arm of chromosome 13.
Ans. **False.** Chromosome 17 at 17q11.1-q12.

20. Cyproheptadine has been associated with weight loss.
Ans. **False.** It is associated with weight gain.

21. Leptin is a peptide that belongs to the interleukin 6 cytokine family.
Ans. **True.**

22. Glycine is an excitatory transmitter in spinal cord.
Ans. **False.** It is inhibitory.

23. Acetazolamide is a carbonic anhydrase inhibitor licensed for use in conjunction with other antiepileptic drugs.
Ans. **True.**

24. Naltrexone is a long acting orally administered μ receptor antagonist.
Ans. **True.** It's half-life is 24 – 72 hours.

25. Dopamine auto receptor antagonists increase both REM and non-REM sleep.
Ans. **False.** They reduce these.

26. Opiate antagonists are associated with short-term reduction in binge eating.
Ans. **True.**

27. Alpha2 adrenoceptor antagonists have shown efficacy in improving memory in schizophrenic patients.
Ans. **True.**

28. Receptors are protein molecules synthesized in the cell body of the neuron.
Ans. **True.**

29. Nausea and vomiting are major side effects of ergolines (bromocriptine, lisuride and pergolide).
Ans. **True.**

30. Desmopressin has shown efficacy in reducing the frequency of the enuresis at night.
Ans. **True.**

31. Concurrent administration of lithium with an SSRI can result in serotonin syndrome.
Ans. **True.**

32. Valproic acid increases slow wave sleep in adults but decreases it in children.
Ans. **False.** The opposite is true.

33. Low Ki value of a drug reflects its greater affinity for the receptor.
Ans. **True.**

34. Stimulation of the κ receptors generates reinforcing properties.
Ans. **False.**

35. Rivastigmine is a pseudo-irreversible inhibitor of both acetyl and butyryl cholinesterases.
Ans. **True.**

36. Clonidine worsens the severity of tics in persons with tic disorder and comorbid ADHD.
Ans. **False.** Reduces.

37. S-demethylcitalopram is the main metabolite of escitalopram.
Ans. **True.**

38. Symptoms of anticholinergic intoxication include mydriasis.

Ans. True.

39. Lithium reduces the functional activity of postsynaptic beta receptors.
Ans. True.

40. Mirtazapine acts as an antagonist of histamine H_1 receptors.
Ans. True.

41. MAOIs should be discontinued at least two weeks before starting carbamazepine treatment.
Ans. True.

42. Fluoxetine induces elevated mood in non-depressed healthy individuals.
Ans. False.

43. Drugs which lower serum amylase levels include valproate.
Ans. False. Valproate raises amylase levels.

44. Opioids are derivatives of the naturally occurring compound opium.
Ans. False. Opioids are synthetic narcotics.

45. Hypnotic drugs decrease stage 1 of non-REM sleep and prolong stage 2 sleep.
Ans. True.

46. Tolerance of the tuberoinfundibular dopaminergic system to the action of neuroleptics does not develop.
Ans. True.

47. The low incidence of side effects with SSRIs is due to their lack of antihistaminergic and anti $-\alpha_1$ adrenergic receptor activities.
Ans. True.

48. Increased fat to lean body mass ratio is associated with decrease in the half-lives of lipophilic drugs.
Ans. False. It is associated with an increase in their half-lives.

49. Flumazenil reverses the anticonvulsant effect of clonazepam.
Ans. True.

50. Venlafaxine is a bicyclic phenyl ethylamine derivative.
Ans. True.

Paper 28

		True	False
1.	Bromocriptine acts as a partial agonist at D_1 receptors and a full agonist at D_2 receptors.	☐	☐
2.	Plasma protein binding of escitalopram is higher than that of other SSRIs.	☐	☐
3.	Phenytoin decreases REM sleep and increases stage 4 sleep.	☐	☐
4.	Deficits in latent inhibition in patients with schizophrenia are reduced by both typical and atypical anti psychotic drugs.	☐	☐
5.	Cataplexy is reduced by drugs that increase signalling by blocking the norepinephrine transporter.	☐	☐
6.	Body Mass Index (BMI) is calculated by dividing a person's weight in kilograms by the square of his or her height in feet.	☐	☐
7.	Norepinephrine firing rate is increased in acute opioid intoxication.	☐	☐
8.	Carbamazepine induced decrease in white cell count can be reversed by the coadministration of lithium.	☐	☐
9.	Antipsychotic dose equivalents are well established among atypical antipsychotic drugs.	☐	☐
10.	Affinity of an antipsychotic drug is dependent on the rates of its association and dissociation with the receptor.	☐	☐
11.	Atomoxetine is not recommended in patients with narrow angle glaucoma.	☐	☐
12.	There is significant difference in efficacy against positive and negative symptoms between different atypical antipsychotic drugs.	☐	☐
13.	Experimental studies have shown that benzodiazepine inverse agonists have cognitive enhancing effects.	☐	☐
14.	Aldosterone synthesis is decreased following chronic lithium treatment.	☐	☐
15.	Modafinil is metabolised by CYP2C9.	☐	☐
16.	In drug development, both animal and human preclinical models are equally constrained by ethical issues.	☐	☐
17.	The tyramine pressor test and the dorsal hand vein constrictor tests are used to establish the dose at which venlafaxine produces norepinephrine reuptake inhibition.	☐	☐
18.	Coadministration of modafinil and phenytoin may lead to phenytoin toxicity.	☐	☐
19.	Valproate shows linear protein binding.	☐	☐
20.	Both cocaine and amphetamine block the reuptake of both norepinephrine and serotonin.	☐	☐
21.	Bretazenil is a long-acting tetracyclic 2,4 benzodiazepine.	☐	☐
22.	Guanfacine is an α_2 – adrenergic receptor antagonist.	☐	☐
23.	Trazodone does not decrease stage 4 sleep.	☐	☐

24. O-desmethylvenlafaxine, an active metabolite of venlafaxine, has monoamine-oxidase B inhibitory activity.　☐　☐

25. The affinity of haloperidol for the D_4 receptor is higher than that of olanzapine.　☐　☐

26. Dehydro-aripiprazole is the active metabolite of aripiprazole.　☐　☐

27. Alcohol decreases the release of opioid peptides in vivo.　☐　☐

28. Phencyclidine (PCP) antagonizes the N-methyl-D-aspartate (NMDA) receptor.　☐　☐

29. Aspirin can enhance the efficacy and toxicity of valproate.　☐　☐

30. The anorexigenic effects of sympathomimetic drugs gradually increase after a few weeks of use.　☐　☐

31. Carbamazepine increases slow-wave sleep and suppresses REM sleep.　☐　☐

32. Approach / avoidance conflict tests have shown that anxiolytic drugs increase approach behaviour.　☐　☐

33. Haemodialysis is likely to be useful in overdose management of the drugs which are highly bound to plasma proteins.　☐　☐

34. Acamprosate is a synthetic indirect GABA antagonist.　☐　☐

35. Elderly patients are more prone than younger ones to develop anticholinergic drug induced toxic confusional states.　☐　☐

36. 4-hydroxyatomoxetine is equipotent to atomoxetine as an inhibitor of the presynaptic noradrenaline transporter.　☐　☐

37. Major metabolic pathways of valproate elimination include glucuronide conjugation but not mitochondrial β -oxidation.　☐　☐

38. Corticotropin Releasing Hormone (CRH) produces symptoms of depression and anxiety by activation of the CRH_1 receptors.　☐　☐

39. The serotonin 1A receptor (HTR1A) gene is located on X chromosome.　☐　☐

40. 5 – 15% of elderly people who have never received neuroleptics manifest an orofacial dyskinesia.　☐　☐

41. There is no correlation between serum lithium levels and responsiveness of depressive symptoms to lithium augmentation of antidepressants.　☐　☐

42. Headache is a rare side-effect of modafinil.　☐　☐

43. GABA is degraded by the enzyme GABA transaminase (GABA-T) to succinic semialdehyde.　☐　☐

44. The greater the protein binding of a medication, the lower the dose required in renal failure.　☐　☐

45. Carbamazepine has been reported to cause hypernatraemia.　☐　☐

46. Clonidine – methylphenidate combination can result in sudden death in children.　☐　☐

47. Carbamazepine decreases atrioventricular conduction.　☐　☐

	True	False

48. Naltrexone has a longer half-life than its major metabolite 6-β-naltrexol. ☐ ☐

49. Platelets can be used as peripheral models of central neurotransmission. ☐ ☐

50. Clozapine clearance is lower in ageing women than men because of low levels of isoenzyme CYP3A4 in women. ☐ ☐

Paper 28

1. **Bromocriptine acts as a partial agonist at D_1 receptors and a full agonist at D_2 receptors.**
Ans. True.

2. **Plasma protein binding of escitalopram is higher than that of other SSRIs.**
Ans. False. It is lower.

3. **Phenytoin decreases REM sleep and increases stage 4 sleep.**
Ans. True.

4. **Deficits in latent inhibition in patients with schizophrenia are reduced by both typical and atypical anti psychotic drugs.**
Ans. True.

5. **Cataplexy is reduced by drugs that increase signalling by blocking the norepinephrine transporter.**
Ans. True.

6. **Body Mass Index (BMI) is calculated by dividing a person's weight in kilograms by the square of his or her height in feet.**
Ans. False. Height is measured in meters.

7. **Norepinephrine firing rate is increased in acute opioid intoxication.**
Ans. False. It is decreased.

8. **Carbamazepine induced decrease in white cell count can be reversed by the coadministration of lithium.**
Ans. True.

9. **Antipsychotic dose equivalents are well established among atypical antipsychotic drugs.**
Ans. False.

10. **Affinity of an antipsychotic drug is dependent on the rates of its association and dissociation with the receptor.**
Ans. True.

11. **Atomoxetine is not recommended in patients with narrow angle glaucoma.**
Ans. True.

12. **There is significant difference in efficacy against positive and negative symptoms between different atypical antipsychotic drugs.**
Ans. False. There is no proven difference.

13. **Experimental studies have shown that benzodiazepine inverse agonists have cognitive enhancing effects.**
Ans. True.

14. **Aldosterone synthesis is decreased following chronic lithium treatment.**
Ans. False. It is increased.

15. **Modafinil is metabolised by CYP2C9.**
Ans. True.

16. **In drug development, both animal and human preclinical models are equally constrained by ethical issues.**
Ans. False. Human models are more constrained.

17. **The tyramine pressor test and the dorsal hand vein constrictor tests are used to establish the dose at which venlafaxine produces norepinephrine reuptake inhibition.**
Ans. True.

18. Coadministration of modafinil and phenytoin may lead to phenytoin toxicity.
Ans. True.

19. Valproate shows linear protein binding.
Ans. False. It shows non-linear protein binding.

20. Both cocaine and amphetamine block the reuptake of both norepinephrine and serotonin.
Ans. True.

21. Bretazenil is a long-acting tetracyclic 2,4 benzodiazepine.
Ans. True.

22. Guanfacine is an α_2 – adrenergic receptor antagonist.
Ans. False. It is an agonist.

23. Trazodone does not decrease stage 4 sleep.
Ans. True.

24. O-desmethylvenlafaxine, an active metabolite of venlafaxine, has monoamine-oxidase B inhibitory activity.
Ans. False.

25. The affinity of haloperidol for the D_4 receptor is higher than that of olanzapine.
Ans. True.

26. Dehydro-aripiprazole is the active metabolite of aripiprazole.
Ans. True.

27. Alcohol decreases the release of opioid peptides in vivo.
Ans. False. It increases this.

28. Phencyclidine (PCP) antagonizes the N-methyl-D-aspartate (NMDA) receptor.
Ans. True.

29. Aspirin can enhance the efficacy and toxicity of valproate.
Ans. True. By displacing it from the plasma proteins.

30. The anorexigenic effects of sympathomimetic drugs gradually increase after a few weeks of use.
Ans. False. They decrease.

31. Carbamazepine increases slow-wave sleep and suppresses REM sleep.
Ans. True.

32. Approach / avoidance conflict tests have shown that anxiolytic drugs increase approach behaviour.
Ans. True.

33. Haemodialysis is likely to be useful in overdose management of the drugs which are highly bound to plasma proteins.
Ans. False. It is unlikely to be useful.

34. Acamprosate is a synthetic indirect GABA antagonist.
Ans. False. It is a GABA agonist.

35. Elderly patients are more prone than younger ones to develop anticholinergic drug induced toxic confusional states.
Ans. True.

36. 4-hydroxyatomoxetine is equipotent to atomoxetine as an inhibitor of the presynaptic noradrenaline transporter.
Ans. True.

37. Major metabolic pathways of valproate elimination include glucuronide conjugation but not mitochondrial β -oxidation.

Ans. **False.** Both are major metabolic pathways.

38. Corticotropin Releasing Hormone (CRH) produces symptoms of depression and anxiety by activation of the CRH_1 receptors.

Ans. **True.**

39. The serotonin 1A receptor (HTR1A) gene is located on X chromosome.

Ans. **False.** Chromosome 5 at 5q11.2-q13.

40. 5 – 15% of elderly people who have never received neuroleptics manifest an orofacial dyskinesia.

Ans. **True.**

41. There is no correlation between serum lithium levels and responsiveness of depressive symptoms to lithium augmentation of antidepressants.

Ans. **True.**

42. Headache is a rare side-effect of modafinil.

Ans. **False.** It is very common.

43. GABA is degraded by the enzyme GABA transaminase (GABA-T) to succinic semialdehyde.

Ans. **True.**

44. The greater the protein binding of a medication, the lower the dose required in renal failure.

Ans. **True.**

45. Carbamazepine has been reported to cause hypernatraemia.

Ans. **False.** It can cause hyponatraemia.

46. Clonidine – methylphenidate combination can result in sudden death in children.

Ans. **True.**

47. Carbamazepine decreases atrioventricular conduction.

Ans. **True.**

48. Naltrexone has a longer half-life than its major metabolite 6-β-naltrexol.

Ans. **False.** It is shorter, 4 hours.

49. Platelets can be used as peripheral models of central neurotransmission.

Ans. **True.**

50. Clozapine clearance is lower in ageing women than men because of low levels of isoenzyme CYP3A4 in women.

Ans. **True.**

Paper 29

	True	False
1. Diffusion rate of a drug is inversely proportional to the concentration gradient across a membrane.	☐	☐
2. Age has been identified as a risk factor for clozapine induced agranulocytosis.	☐	☐
3. The CB_2 is the central cannabinoid receptor that binds 11-hydroxy-tetrahydrocannabinol.	☐	☐
4. Apomorphine-stimulated growth hormone secretion is lower in untreated patients with schizophrenia.	☐	☐
5. Mirtazapine can increase both serum cholesterol and triglycerides.	☐	☐
6. The Yale-Brown Obsessive-Compulsive Scale (Y-BOCS) can be used to assess the response to drug treatment in obsessive compulsive disorder.	☐	☐
7. The Abnormal Involuntary Movement Scale (AIMS) allows rating of abnormal movements by the patient.	☐	☐
8. The serotonin 2A receptor (HTR2A) gene is located on chromosome 13 at 13q14-q21.	☐	☐
9. Neuroleptic malignant syndrome has been associated with antipsychotic drug switches.	☐	☐
10. The use of nonsteroidal anti-inflammatory drugs (NSAIDs) well before the onset of the Alzheimer's disease has been associated with a decreased incidence of Alzheimer's disease in old age.	☐	☐
11. Anticholinergic drugs can worsen tardive dyskinesia but not tardive dystonia.	☐	☐
12. Binding of tricyclic antidepressants to brain proteins is smaller than to plasma proteins.	☐	☐
13. Clozapine reduces the exacerbation of symptoms in schizophrenic patients given ketamine.	☐	☐
14. Concurrent use of SSRIs with ECT has been reported to prolong the seizures.	☐	☐
15. Phase I oxidative metabolic pathways are more prone to induction or inhibition than are the Phase II type pathways.	☐	☐
16. Gabapentin undergoes hepatic metabolism.	☐	☐
17. Medroxyprogesterone acetate increases the metabolic clearance of testosterone.	☐	☐
18. The longer the half-life of a drug, the greater the volume of its distribution.	☐	☐
19. Distribution of a drug from blood to brain occurs slower than from blood to peripheral fatty tissue.	☐	☐
20. Cyproterone acetate blocks intracellular testosterone uptake at the androgen receptors.	☐	☐
21. The incidence of major teratogenic effects associated with maternal antiepileptic drug use is 0.5%.	☐	☐
22. Nabilone is a synthetic cannabinoid with anti-emetic properties used for the treatment of nausea and vomiting caused by cytotoxic chemotherapy.	☐	☐

23. Tolerance to the psychological effects of LSD develops slowly. ☐ ☐

24. Yohimbine blocks the pharmacological effects of clonidine. ☐ ☐

25. Use of folic acid during pregnancy in all women taking valproate has been shown to reduce the risk of neural tube defects. ☐ ☐

26. Learning disability is a contraindication to antiepileptic drug withdrawal. ☐ ☐

27. Drugs with high affinity for the adipose tissue will have faster elimination in women than in men. ☐ ☐

28. A surrogate biomarker can act as a substitute for a clinical outcome measure. ☐ ☐

29. When receptor occupancy results in less than the maximal effect of the endogenous ligand the drug is said to be a partial agonist. ☐ ☐

30. Inhibition of glycogen synthase kinase 3 beta (GSK – 3Beta) has been implicated in the mediation of lithium's acute effects. ☐ ☐

31. Potassium sparing and osmotic diuretics are known to increase serum lithium concentration. ☐ ☐

32. Grapefruit juice decreases the bioavailability of drugs that are metabolised by CYP3A4 and CYP1A2. ☐ ☐

33. LSD does not cause physical dependence. ☐ ☐

34. SSRIs have been reported to increase the risk of neurocardiogenic symptoms. ☐ ☐

35. The response to thyroid hormone supplementation of antidepressants is correlated with the laboratory measures of thyroid function. ☐ ☐

36. The biodistribution of the drug can be studied by radio-labelling of the drug but not its derivatives. ☐ ☐

37. The mean clearance of Quetiapine in elderly patients is lower than in healthy adults. ☐ ☐

38. The activity of drug-metabolizing enzymes can be described by the Michaelin-Menten equation. ☐ ☐

39. The hydrolysis reactions of a drug's metabolism are mediated by nonmicrosomal enzymes. ☐ ☐

40. Both clonidine and guanfacine should be avoided in adults with a blood pressure below 90/60 mm Hg. ☐ ☐

41. The extent of drug binding to plasma proteins is higher in neonates than in adults. ☐ ☐

42. Reduction in active transport in elderly is of little clinical importance for psychotropic drugs. ☐ ☐

43. Concomitant use of lithium and carbamazepine is recommended in the treatment of patients with bipolar disorder and comorbid CNS disease. ☐ ☐

44. Pharmacokinetic interactions occur when a drug alters what the patient's physiology does to another drug. ☐ ☐

45. The fluctuating course of psychiatric disorders increase the number of patients experiencing a placebo effect. ☐ ☐

46. Chronic benzodiazepine abuse inhibits the expression of mRNA coding for the α_1 subunit of GABA$_A$ receptor.   ☐   ☐

47. SSRIs are associated with a self-limiting neonatal withdrawal syndrome.   ☐   ☐

48. The withdrawal of antiepileptic drugs in patients with symptomatic epilepsy is more likely to be successful than in patients with idiopathic epilepsy.   ☐   ☐

49. Concurrent treatment with lithium and valproate can increase the risk of developing additive adverse reactions such as sedation, weight gain and tremor.   ☐   ☐

50. Hepatic clearance is the product of hepatic extraction ratio and hepatic blood flow.   ☐   ☐

Paper 29

1. Diffusion rate of a drug is inversely proportional to the concentration gradient across a membrane.
Ans. **False.** They are directly proportional.

2. Age has been identified as a risk factor for clozapine induced agranulocytosis.
Ans. **False.**

3. The CB_2 is the central cannabinoid receptor that binds 11-hydroxy-tetrahydrocannabinol.
Ans. **False.** CB_1 is.

4. Apomorphine-stimulated growth hormone secretion is lower in untreated patients with schizophrenia.
Ans. **False.** It is higher in these patients.

5. Mirtazapine can increase both serum cholesterol and triglycerides.
Ans. **True.**

6. The Yale-Brown Obsessive-Compulsive Scale (Y-BOCS) can be used to assess the response to drug treatment in obsessive compulsive disorder.
Ans. **True.**

7. The Abnormal Involuntary Movement Scale (AIMS) allows rating of abnormal movements by the patient.
Ans. **False.** It is rated by the clinician.

8. The serotonin 2A receptor (HTR2A) gene is located on chromosome 13 at 13q14-q21.
Ans. **True.**

9. Neuroleptic malignant syndrome has been associated with antipsychotic drug switches.
Ans. **True.**

10. The use of nonsteroidal anti-inflammatory drugs (NSAIDs) well before the onset of the Alzheimer's disease has been associated with a decreased incidence of Alzheimer's disease in old age.
Ans. **True.**

11. Anticholinergic drugs can worsen tardive dyskinesia but not tardive dystonia.
Ans. **True.**

12. Binding of tricyclic antidepressants to brain proteins is smaller than to plasma proteins.
Ans. **False.** It is greater.

13. Clozapine reduces the exacerbation of symptoms in schizophrenic patients given ketamine.
Ans. **True.**

14. Concurrent use of SSRIs with ECT has been reported to prolong the seizures.
Ans. **True.**

15. Phase I oxidative metabolic pathways are more prone to induction or inhibition than are the Phase II type pathways.
Ans. **True.**

16. Gabapentin undergoes hepatic metabolism.
Ans. **False.** It is excreted unchanged.

17. Medroxyprogesterone acetate increases the metabolic clearance of testosterone.
Ans. **True.**

18. The longer the half-life of a drug, the greater the volume of its distribution.
Ans. **True.**

19. Distribution of a drug from blood to brain occurs slower than from blood to peripheral fatty tissue.
Ans. False. Quicker.

20. Cyproterone acetate blocks intracellular testosterone uptake at the androgen receptors.
Ans. True.

21. The incidence of major teratogenic effects associated with maternal antiepileptic drug use is 0.5%.
Ans. False. 4 – 6%.

22. Nabilone is a synthetic cannabinoid with anti-emetic properties used for the treatment of nausea and vomiting caused by cytotoxic chemotherapy.
Ans. True.

23. Tolerance to the psychological effects of LSD develops slowly.
Ans. False. Rapidly (2 – 4 days).

24. Yohimbine blocks the pharmacological effects of clonidine.
Ans. True.

25. Use of folic acid during pregnancy in all women taking valproate has been shown to reduce the risk of neural tube defects.
Ans. True.

26. Learning disability is a contraindication to antiepileptic drug withdrawal.
Ans. False.

27. Drugs with high affinity for the adipose tissue will have faster elimination in women than in men.
Ans. False. Elimination is slower in women than in men.

28. A surrogate biomarker can act as a substitute for a clinical outcome measure.
Ans. True.

29. When receptor occupancy results in less than the maximal effect of the endogenous ligand the drug is said to be a partial agonist.
Ans. True.

30. Inhibition of glycogen synthase kinase 3 beta (GSK – 3Beta) has been implicated in the mediation of lithium's acute effects.
Ans. True.

31. Potassium sparing and osmotic diuretics are known to increase serum lithium concentration.
Ans. False. Decrease.

32. Grapefruit juice decreases the bioavailability of drugs that are metabolised by CYP3A4 and CYP1A2.
Ans. False. It increases it by inhibiting the enzymes.

33. LSD does not cause physical dependence.
Ans. True.

34. SSRIs have been reported to increase the risk of neurocardiogenic symptoms.
Ans. False. They reduce this.

35. The response to thyroid hormone supplementation of antidepressants is correlated with the laboratory measures of thyroid function.
Ans. False.

36. The biodistribution of the drug can be studied by radio-labelling of the drug but not its derivatives.
Ans. False. Either drug or its derivatives can be radiolabelled.

37. The mean clearance of Quetiapine in elderly patients is lower than in healthy adults.
Ans. True.

38. The activity of drug-metabolizing enzymes can be described by the Michaelin-Menten equation.
Ans. True.

39. The hydrolysis reactions of a drug's metabolism are mediated by nonmicrosomal enzymes.
Ans. True.

40. Both clonidine and guanfacine should be avoided in adults with a blood pressure below 90/60 mm Hg.
Ans. True.

41. The extent of drug binding to plasma proteins is higher in neonates than in adults.
Ans. False. Lower.

42. Reduction in active transport in elderly is of little clinical importance for psychotropic drugs.
Ans. True. They are absorbed by passive diffusion.

43. Concomitant use of lithium and carbamazepine is recommended in the treatment of patients with bipolar disorder and comorbid CNS disease.
Ans. False. It carries an increased risk of neurotoxicity.

44. Pharmacokinetic interactions occur when a drug alters what the patient's physiology does to another drug.
Ans. True.

45. The fluctuating course of psychiatric disorders increase the number of patients experiencing a placebo effect.
Ans. True.

46. Chronic benzodiazepine abuse inhibits the expression of mRNA coding for the α_1 subunit of GABA$_A$ receptor.
Ans. True.

47. SSRIs are associated with a self-limiting neonatal withdrawal syndrome.
Ans. True.

48. The withdrawal of antiepileptic drugs in patients with symptomatic epilepsy is more likely to be successful than in patients with idiopathic epilepsy.
Ans. False. Less likely to be successful.

49. Concurrent treatment with lithium and valproate can increase the risk of developing additive adverse reactions such as sedation, weight gain and tremor.
Ans. True.

50. Hepatic clearance is the product of hepatic extraction ratio and hepatic blood flow.
Ans. True.

Paper 30

		True	False

1. Fluoxetine and paroxetine reduce the hypotensive effect of metoprolol. ☐ ☐

2. Provided the same amount of a drug has entered the plasma, the area under the concentration time curve (AUC) is the same irrespective of the route of administration. ☐ ☐

3. Clonidine inhibits the increased activity in the locus coeruleus and suppresses the opiate-withdrawal symptoms. ☐ ☐

4. Past history of neuroleptic malignant syndrome is an absolute contraindication for subsequent therapy with dopamine antagonists. ☐ ☐

5. $GABA_A$ and $GABA_C$ receptors are ionotropic receptors, and $GABA_B$ is a metabotropic receptor. ☐ ☐

6. Partial dopamine receptor agonists may behave like agonists at autoreceptors and act as antagonists at post synaptic receptors. ☐ ☐

7. Apomorphine-stimulated growth hormone secretion is reported to be blunted following both acute and chronic neuroleptic treatment. ☐ ☐

8. Carbamazepine induced idiosyncratic adverse effects include blurred vision. ☐ ☐

9. Cocaine has high affinity for the dopamine transporter. ☐ ☐

10. Modafinil selectively decreases neuronal activation in the hypothalamus. ☐ ☐

11. Age-associated reduction in splanchnic blood flow is associated with reduction in absorption of lipophilic drugs. ☐ ☐

12. Paroxetine causes less sexual side-effects than fluvoxamine. ☐ ☐

13. Voluntary intoxication may present as a legal defence if the offence requires the presence of a specific intent. ☐ ☐

14. Bioavailability of an orally administered drug equals unity. ☐ ☐

15. Neuroleptic malignant syndrome has been reported in patients with Parkinson's disease whose dopaminergic treatment is withdrawn. ☐ ☐

16. 90% of the body's supply of serotonin is in the CNS. ☐ ☐

17. Tiagabine is a selective GABA reuptake inhibitor with high selectivity for the GABA transporter GAT – 1. ☐ ☐

18. Smoking reduces the half-life and increases the clearance of olanzapine. ☐ ☐

19. Maintenance treatment with antidepressant drugs to prevent recurrences should continue for 12 weeks. ☐ ☐

20. The SSRIs are effective for treatment of panic disorder with or without agoraphobia ☐ ☐

21. A minimum of 6 months seizure-free period is required before considering antiepileptic drug withdrawal to reduce the chance of relapse. ☐ ☐

22. Pharmacodynamic interactions occur when a drug alters what another drug does to a patients physiology. ☐ ☐

23. SSRIs have been shown to increase the risk of gastrointestinal bleeding in the elderly. ☐ ☐

24. Intoxication can be held as involuntary if it is caused by prescribed drugs taken according to instructions. ☐ ☐

25. The risk of drug rash is higher with valproic acid than with carbamazepine after the first two months of use. ☐ ☐

26. Aging is associated with reduction in the volume of distribution for water-soluble drugs. ☐ ☐

27. Tricyclic antidepressants have been shown to increase serum glucose levels significantly. ☐ ☐

28. Citalopram is a strong inhibitor of CYP2D6. ☐ ☐

29. Family history of QTc prolongation is a risk factor for antipsychotic-induced QTc prolongation. ☐ ☐

30. Topiramate induced weight loss has been reported to be dose related. ☐ ☐

31. SSRIs have shown efficacy in the treatment of PTSD without comorbid depression. ☐ ☐

32. SSRIs do not raise plasma serotonin concentrations. ☐ ☐

33. Methylxanthines (eg. caffeine, theophylline) decrease renal lithium clearance. ☐ ☐

34. Fluoxetine has been shown to cause hypoglycaemia in non-insulin dependent diabetes. ☐ ☐

35. Patients with schizophrenia are likely to respond to smaller doses of antipsychotic drugs if they are heavy cigarette smokers. ☐ ☐

36. CYP2D6 metabolism occurs both in the brain and in the liver. ☐ ☐

37. Norfluoxetine is a potent CYP3A4 inhibitor unlike fluoxetine which is a weak inhibitor. ☐ ☐

38. The bioavailability of a drug calculated with reference to an intravenous dose is its relative bioavailability. ☐ ☐

39. The overall prevalence of prescribed stimulant drug use in children has been estimated as higher in Britain than in the USA ☐ ☐

40. People with first-episode psychosis are more sensitive to neuroleptic induced extrapyramidal side-effects. ☐ ☐

41. If depressive symptoms return during the continuation period with antidepressant therapy, it is considered to be a recurrence. ☐ ☐

42. Effective antidepressant treatment normalizes the elevated corticotrophin-releasing factor levels in CSF of depressed patients. ☐ ☐

43. 1-pyramidnyl/piperazine (1-PP) is an active metabolite of buspirone. ☐ ☐

44. Increased body fat is associated with longer half-life of the drugs. ☐ ☐

45. Clonazepam is effective in controlling both the behavioural and the dream-disordered components of REM sleep behaviour disorder. ☐ ☐

46. Approximately 75% of patients with major depression show a blunted thyroid-stimulating hormone response to thyrotrophin-releasing hormone. ☐   ☐

47. After achieving steady state in plasma, a drug's steady state concentration is dependent on the volume of distribution. ☐   ☐

48. Stimulants are effective in the short to medium term in reducing the core symptoms of ADHD. ☐   ☐

49. Impulsivity has been correlated with a high platelet MAO activity. ☐   ☐

50. Gonadotrophin-releasing hormone stimulation test is a very sensitive test of hypothalamic-pituitary-gonadal axis activity. ☐   ☐

Paper 30

1. **Fluoxetine and paroxetine reduce the hypotensive effect of metoprolol.**
Ans. **False.** They enhance it by inhibiting CYP2D6.

2. **Provided the same amount of a drug has entered the plasma, the area under the concentration time curve (AUC) is the same irrespective of the route of administration.**
Ans. **True.**

3. **Clonidine inhibits the increased activity in the locus coeruleus and suppresses the opiate-withdrawal symptoms.**
Ans. **True.**

4. **Past history of neuroleptic malignant syndrome is an absolute contraindication for subsequent therapy with dopamine antagonists.**
Ans. **False.** High potency antipsychotics should be avoided.

5. **$GABA_A$ and $GABA_C$ receptors are ionotropic receptors, and $GABA_B$ is a metabotropic receptor.**
Ans. **True.**

6. **Partial dopamine receptor agonists may behave like agonists at autoreceptors and act as antagonists at post synaptic receptors.**
Ans. **True.**

7. **Apomorphine-stimulated growth hormone secretion is reported to be blunted following both acute and chronic neuroleptic treatment.**
Ans. **True.**

8. **Carbamazepine induced idiosyncratic adverse effects include blurred vision.**
Ans. **False.** It is a dose related effect.

9. **Cocaine has high affinity for the dopamine transporter.**
Ans. **True.**

10. **Modafinil selectively decreases neuronal activation in the hypothalamus.**
Ans. **False.** Increases.

11. **Age-associated reduction in splanchnic blood flow is associated with reduction in absorption of lipophilic drugs.**
Ans. **True.**

12. **Paroxetine causes less sexual side-effects than fluvoxamine.**
A **False.** The opposite is true.

13. **Voluntary intoxication may present as a legal defence if the offence requires the presence of a specific intent.**
Ans. **True.**

14. **Bioavailability of an orally administered drug equals unity.**
Ans. **False.** It is always less than unity.

15. **Neuroleptic malignant syndrome has been reported in patients with Parkinson's disease whose dopaminergic treatment is withdrawn.**
Ans. **True.**

16. **90% of the body's supply of serotonin is in the CNS.**
Ans. **False.** CNS (2%), Gut (90%), Platelets (8%).

17. **Tiagabine is a selective GABA reuptake inhibitor with high selectivity for the GABA transporter GAT – 1.**
Ans. **True.**

18. Smoking reduces the half-life and increases the clearance of olanzapine.
Ans. True.

19. Maintenance treatment with antidepressant drugs to prevent recurrences should continue for 12 weeks.
Ans. False. Treatment should be > 1 year.

20. The SSRIs are effective for treatment of panic disorder with or without agoraphobia
Ans. True.

21. A minimum of 6 months seizure-free period is required before considering antiepileptic drug withdrawal to reduce the chance of relapse.
Ans. False. It can be considered after a minimum of 2 years.

22. Pharmacodynamic interactions occur when a drug alters what another drug does to a patients physiology.
Ans. True.

23. SSRIs have been shown to increase the risk of gastrointestinal bleeding in the elderly.
Ans. True.

24. Intoxication can be held as involuntary if it is caused by prescribed drugs taken according to instructions.
Ans. True.

25. The risk of drug rash is higher with valproic acid than with carbamazepine after the first two months of use.
Ans. False. Higher with carbamazepine.

26. Aging is associated with reduction in the volume of distribution for water-soluble drugs.
Ans. True.

27. Tricyclic antidepressants have been shown to increase serum glucose levels significantly.
Ans. True.

28. Citalopram is a strong inhibitor of CYP2D6.
Ans. False. It is a weak inhibitor.

29. Family history of QTc prolongation is a risk factor for antipsychotic-induced QTc prolongation.
Ans. True.

30. Topiramate induced weight loss has been reported to be dose related.
Ans. True.

31. SSRIs have shown efficacy in the treatment of PTSD without comorbid depression.
Ans. True.

32. SSRIs do not raise plasma serotonin concentrations.
Ans. True.

33. Methylxanthines (eg. caffeine, theophylline) decrease renal lithium clearance.
Ans. False. They increase it.

34. Fluoxetine has been shown to cause hypoglycaemia in non-insulin dependent diabetes.
Ans. True.

35. Patients with schizophrenia are likely to respond to smaller doses of antipsychotic drugs if they are heavy cigarette smokers.
Ans. False. The opposite is true.

36. CYP2D6 metabolism occurs both in the brain and in the liver.
Ans. True.

37. **Norfluoxetine is a potent CYP3A4 inhibitor unlike fluoxetine which is a weak inhibitor.**

Ans. **True.**

38. **The bioavailability of a drug calculated with reference to an intravenous dose is its relative bioavailability.**

Ans. **False.** Absolute bioavailability.

39. **The overall prevalence of prescribed stimulant drug use in children has been estimated as higher in Britain than in the USA**

Ans. **False.** It is higher in the USA.

40. **People with first-episode psychosis are more sensitive to neuroleptic induced extrapyramidal side-effects.**

Ans. **True.**

41. **If depressive symptoms return during the continuation period with antidepressant therapy, it is considered to be a recurrence.**

Ans. **False.** Relapse.

42. **Effective antidepressant treatment normalizes the elevated corticotrophin-releasing factor levels in CSF of depressed patients.**

Ans. **True.**

43. **1-pyramidnyl/piperazine (1-PP) is an active metabolite of buspirone.**

Ans. **True.**

44. **Increased body fat is associated with longer half-life of the drugs.**

Ans. **True.**

45. **Clonazepam is effective in controlling both the behavioural and the dream-disordered components of REM sleep behaviour disorder.**

Ans. **True.**

46. **Approximately 75% of patients with major depression show a blunted thyroid-stimulating hormone response to thyrotrophin-releasing hormone.**

Ans. **False.** 25% of such patients exhibit this.

47. **After achieving steady state in plasma, a drug's steady state concentration is dependent on the volume of distribution.**

Ans. **False.** They are independent of each other.

48. **Stimulants are effective in the short to medium term in reducing the core symptoms of ADHD.**

Ans. **True.**

49. **Impulsivity has been correlated with a high platelet MAO activity.**

Ans. **False.** Low.

50. **Gonadotrophin-releasing hormone stimulation test is a very sensitive test of hypothalamic-pituitary-gonadal axis activity.**

Ans. **True.**

Paper 31

		True	False
1.	Low prefrontal D_1 receptor density has been associated with poor performance on the Wisconsin card sort test in patients with schizophrenia.	☐	☐
2.	Differences in physicochemical properties are more between diastereomers than between enantiomers.	☐	☐
3.	Risk of relapse is 10 – 15% during the continuation phase of antidepressant therapy.	☐	☐
4.	Caffeine improves restless legs syndrome.	☐	☐
5.	Norepinephrine is converted to epinephrine via phenyl-N-methyltransferase (PNMT).	☐	☐
6.	Response to antipsychotic medication is not 100% despite their adequate D_2 receptor occupancy.	☐	☐
7.	Acute alcohol intake increases hepatic metabolism of coadministered drugs.	☐	☐
8.	Recognised side-effects of lithium maintenance therapy include hyperparathyroidism with hypercalcemia.	☐	☐
9.	Aging is associated with an increase in the volume of distribution for lipophilic psychotropic drugs.	☐	☐
10.	Low urinary MHPG levels predict response to noradrenergic antidepressant drugs.	☐	☐
11.	Neuroleptic-induced expression of FOS protein in the dorsolateral striatum has been proposed to relate to the drug's potential to cause extra pyramidal side effects.	☐	☐
12.	Anabolic steroid abuse can decrease low-density lipoprotein blood levels.	☐	☐
13.	There is no recognized hallucinogen withdrawal state.	☐	☐
14.	Rapid titration of lamotrigine dosage is associated with a risk of toxic epidermal necrolysis.	☐	☐
15.	Paroxetine causes more weight gain than other SSRIs.	☐	☐
16.	Neurokinin antagonists have shown anxiolytic properties in preclinical studies.	☐	☐
17.	REM sleep latency is increased following withdrawal from REM sleep-suppressing drugs.	☐	☐
18.	Benzodiazepines have been shown to antagonize suppression of natural killer cell activity by corticotrophin-releasing factor.	☐	☐
19.	Dronabinol is a synthetic form of tetrahydrocannabinol.	☐	☐
20.	75% of patients on long term lithium treatment for more than 10 years, develop morphological kidney changes.	☐	☐
21.	α-Methylparatyrosine (AMPT) worsens depressive symptoms in patients on noradrenergic antidepressants but not those on SSRIs.	☐	☐
22.	Neuroleptics decrease c-fos expression in the forebrain.	☐	☐
23.	Coadministration of pentazocine and methadone can cause withdrawal symptoms due to partial antagonist effects of pentazocine.	☐	☐

24. Gamma hydroxy butyrate is a naturally occurring transmitter in the brain which increases dopamine levels in the brain. ☐ ☐

25. Polymorphisms in the NAT-2 gene (N-acetyl transferase-2) result in a bimodal distribution of the population into slow acetylators and rapid acetylators. ☐ ☐

26. Cannabinoids produce a dose-related bradycardia. ☐ ☐

27. Venlafaxine is contraindicated in patients taking MAOIs. ☐ ☐

28. Chronic benzodiazepine abuse causes down regulation of the GABAergic receptors. ☐ ☐

29. Prolactin responses to fenfluramine challenge are blunted in depressed patients. ☐ ☐

30. ["C] Flumazenil is used in studying the dopamine receptors by positron-emission tomography. ☐ ☐

31. 5-HT$_{1A}$ receptor agonists and 5-HT$_{2A}$ receptor antagonists produce similar neurochemical and behavioural effects. ☐ ☐

32. Use of lithium near term can cause floppy baby syndrome. ☐ ☐

33. Polymorphisms in the receptor for a drug can determine variability in its pharmacologic effect. ☐ ☐

34. Continuing treatment with antidepressants reduces the odds of depressive relapse in 10% of patients. ☐ ☐

35. SSRIs may worsen the motor symptoms of Parkinson's disease. ☐ ☐

36. Lithium increases slow wave sleep and has a mild REM suppressant effect. ☐ ☐

37. Steady state is achieved when the rate of drug elimination equals the rate of drug delivery into the systemic circulation. ☐ ☐

38. Following the sudden discontinuation of antidepressant therapy on recovery, 10% of patients will experience a relapse of their depressive symptoms. ☐ ☐

39. Antidepressant withdrawal symptoms in the neonate include agitation and irritability. ☐ ☐

40. There is consistent correlation between risperidone dose, prolactin concentration and the occurrence of symptoms of hyperprolactinaemia. ☐ ☐

41. Protein-binding of nitrazepam is more than that of diazepam. ☐ ☐

42. Folic acid treatment prior to conception reduces the risk of neural tube defects due to carbamazepine. ☐ ☐

43. Alcohol stimulates production of proinflammatory cytokines. ☐ ☐

44. Co-administration of lithium and ACE-inhibitors increase the risk of lithium toxicity. ☐ ☐

45. Cannabinoid receptors are not found in the brainstem. ☐ ☐

46. Drug induced neonatal toxicity is commonly due to first trimester exposure to the drug. ☐ ☐

47. Patients with bipolar II illness respond to lithium prophylaxis better than the patients with bipolar I illness. ☐ ☐

48. **Ziprasidone can cause transient prolactin elevation.** ☐ ☐

49. **Tryptophan depletion has been shown to produce a relapse of depression in depressed patients who have responded to SSRIs.** ☐ ☐

50. **Measurement of the plasma level of cardiac troponin levels may be useful in the diagnosis of clozapine induced myocarditis.** ☐ ☐

Paper 31

1. Low prefrontal D_1 receptor density has been associated with poor performance on the Wisconsin card sort test in patients with schizophrenia.
Ans. True.

2. Differences in physicochemical properties are more between diastereomers than between enantiomers.
Ans. True.

3. Risk of relapse is 10 – 15% during the continuation phase of antidepressant therapy.
Ans. True.

4. Caffeine improves restless legs syndrome.
Ans. False. It worsens it.

5. Norepinephrine is converted to epinephrine via phenyl-N-methyltransferase (PNMT).
Ans. True.

6. Response to antipsychotic medication is not 100% despite their adequate D_2 receptor occupancy.
Ans. True.

7. Acute alcohol intake increases hepatic metabolism of coadministered drugs.
Ans. False. It decreases it.

8. Recognised side-effects of lithium maintenance therapy include hyperparathyroidism with hypercalcemia.
Ans. True.

9. Aging is associated with an increase in the volume of distribution for lipophilic psychotropic drugs.
Ans. True.

10. Low urinary MHPG levels predict response to noradrenergic antidepressant drugs.
Ans. True.

11. Neuroleptic-induced expression of FOS protein in the dorsolateral striatum has been proposed to relate to the drug's potential to cause extra pyramidal side-effects.
Ans. True.

12. Anabolic steroid abuse can decrease low-density lipoprotein blood levels.
Ans. False. Increase.

13. There is no recognized hallucinogen withdrawal state.
Ans. True.

14. Rapid titration of lamotrigine dosage is associated with a risk of toxic epidermal necrolysis.
Ans. True.

15. Paroxetine causes more weight gain than other SSRIs.
Ans. True.

16. Neurokinin antagonists have shown anxiolytic properties in preclinical studies.
Ans. True.

17. REM sleep latency is increased following withdrawal from REM sleep-suppressing drugs.
Ans. False. It is reduced.

18. Benzodiazepines have been shown to antagonize suppression of natural killer cell activity by corticotrophin-releasing factor.
Ans. True.

19. Dronabinol is a synthetic form of tetrahydrocannabinol.
Ans. True.

20. 75% of patients on long term lithium treatment for more than 10 years, develop morphological kidney changes.
Ans. False 10% – 20% of patients.

21. α-Methylparatyrosine (AMPT) worsens depressive symptoms in patients on noradrenergic antidepressants but not those on SSRIs.
Ans. True.

22. Neuroleptics decrease c-fos expression in the forebrain.
Ans. False. They increase it.

23. Coadministration of pentazocine and methadone can cause withdrawal symptoms due to partial antagonist effects of pentazocine.
Ans. True.

24. Gamma hydroxy butyrate is a naturally occurring transmitter in the brain which increases dopamine levels in the brain.
Ans. True.

25. Polymorphisms in the NAT-2 gene (N-acetyl transferase-2) result in a bimodal distribution of the population into slow acetylators and rapid acetylators.
Ans. True.

26. Cannabinoids produce a dose-related bradycardia.
Ans. False. The produce a dose related tachycardia.

27. Venlafaxine is contraindicated in patients taking MAOIs.
Ans. True.

28. Chronic benzodiazepine abuse causes down regulation of the GABAergic receptors.
Ans. True.

29. Prolactin responses to fenfluramine challenge are blunted in depressed patients.
Ans. True.

30. ["C] Flumazenil is used in studying the dopamine receptors by positron-emission tomography.
Ans. False. Used in studying the benzodiazepine receptors.

31. 5-HT_{1A} receptor agonists and 5-HT_{2A} receptor antagonists produce similar neurochemical and behavioural effects.
Ans. True.

32. Use of lithium near term can cause floppy baby syndrome.
Ans. True.

33. Polymorphisms in the receptor for a drug can determine variability in its pharmacologic effect.
Ans. True.

34. Continuing treatment with antidepressants reduces the odds of depressive relapse in 10% of patients.
Ans. False. The odds are reduced by 60 – 70%.

35. SSRIs may worsen the motor symptoms of Parkinson's disease.
Ans. True.

36. Lithium increases slow wave sleep and has a mild REM suppressant effect.
Ans. True.

37. Steady state is achieved when the rate of drug elimination equals the rate of drug delivery into the systemic circulation.
Ans. True.

38. Following the sudden discontinuation of antidepressant therapy on recovery, 10% of patients will experience a relapse of their depressive symptoms.
Ans. False. Up to 50% experience this.

39. Antidepressant withdrawal symptoms in the neonate include agitation and irritability.
Ans. True.

40. There is consistent correlation between risperidone dose, prolactin concentration and the occurrence of symptoms of hyperprolactinaemia.
Ans. False.

41. Protein-binding of nitrazepam is more than that of diazepam.
Ans. False. It is less.

42. Folic acid treatment prior to conception reduces the risk of neural tube defects due to carbamazepine.
Ans. True.

43. Alcohol stimulates production of proinflammatory cytokines.
Ans. False. It inhibits this.

44. Co-administration of lithium and ACE-inhibitors increase the risk of lithium toxicity.
Ans. True. This is due to sodium depletion.

45. Cannabinoid receptors are not found in the brainstem.
Ans. True.

46. Drug induced neonatal toxicity is commonly due to first trimester exposure to the drug.
Ans. False. It is commonly due to third trimester exposure.

47. Patients with bipolar II illness respond to lithium prophylaxis better than the patients with bipolar I illness.
Ans. False.

48. Ziprasidone can cause transient prolactin elevation.
Ans. True.

49. Tryptophan depletion has been shown to produce a relapse of depression in depressed patients who have responded to SSRIs.
Ans. True.

50. Measurement of the plasma level of cardiac troponin levels may be useful in the diagnosis of clozapine induced myocarditis.
Ans. True.

Paper 32

1. Randomized controlled trials have good external but poor internal validity.

2. Both 5-hydroxytryptamine and substance P are involved in co-transmission in brainstem and spinal cord.

3. Unlike type B adverse drug reactions, type A reactions are unpredictable.

4. Diazepam is the treatment of choice for prolonged febrile convulsions.

5. The serotonin 2C receptor (HTR2C) gene is located on the long arm of the X chromosome at Xq24.

6. Bioavailability of an intravenously administered drug equals unity.

7. Cannabinoids produce dose-related increase of intra-ocular pressure.

8. Prophylactic folic acid reduces the incidence of neural tube defects due to valproate or carbamazepine.

9. The binding of drugs to plasma proteins is irreversible.

10. Tricyclic antidepressant drugs have Class Ia antiarrhythmic properties.

11. The association between hypothyroidism and the development of rapid cycling course in patients with bipolar I disorder has been shown as independent of the effects of lithium.

12. Serotonin antagonists antagonize the effects of hallucinogens.

13. SSRIs can cause reversible galactorrhea.

14. Relapse rates after ECT are much higher than those after stopping antidepressants.

15. The dose of amisulpride should be reduced if the patient's creatinine clearance is low.

16. The plasma concentration of diazepam for anxiolytic action is more than that for its anticonvulsant action.

17. Recognized side-effects of clonidine include depression.

18. Prophylactic treatment of major depressive disorder with antidepressants is effective in reducing the severity but not the number of recurrences.

19. Dopamine receptor antagonists increase the reinforcing effects of amphetamine and cocaine.

20. Tetrahydrocannabinol increases slow-wave sleep and reduces REM sleep.

21. Chronic alcohol use decreases hepatic metabolism of coadministered drugs.

22. Quetiapine restores prepulse inhibition of acoustic startle response in apomorphine treated rats.

23. Gabapentin is effective for the treatment of neuropathic pain.

24. Synergistic interactions between two drugs prescribed together produce a greater effect than the sum of their individual effects.

25. A more addictive drug should not be used for detoxification of a patient from a less addictive one. ☐ ☐

26. Alcohol reduces natural killer cell activity and suppresses B- and T-cell immunity. ☐ ☐

27. In vitro $5\text{-HT}_{2A}/D_2$ receptor affinity ratio of ziprasidone is lower than that of most other antipsychotic drugs. ☐ ☐

28. Noradrenaline is a physiological antagonist for acetylcholine. ☐ ☐

29. Common side effects of pseudoephedrine include hallucinations. ☐ ☐

30. Patients with cyclothymic disorder are more likely to develop antidepressant-induced hypomania. ☐ ☐

31. Drug induced tremors are rarely resting tremors. ☐ ☐

32. Both the dissociation constant of the drug and the pH of its solution determine the extent to which a drug is ionised. ☐ ☐

33. Predictors of good antimanic response to lithium include substance misuse. ☐ ☐

34. Examples of two neurotransmitters involved together in cotransmission include GABA and glycine in the cerebellum. ☐ ☐

35. Inhibition caused by drugs occurs slower than enzyme induction. ☐ ☐

36. Alcohol is one of the commonest causes of atrial fibrillation. ☐ ☐

37. 5HT_1 agonists are effective in the treatment of acute migraine attacks. ☐ ☐

38. Pharmaceutical interactions between two drugs occur during their metabolism. ☐ ☐

39. Buspirone has been associated with extrapyramidal side-effects. ☐ ☐

40. Randomized controlled trials of a drug are more generalizable than pragmatic trials. ☐ ☐

41. Adenylyl cyclase and phospholipase C are regulated by G proteins. ☐ ☐

42. The CNS depressant actions of the benzodiazepines and alcohol are additive. ☐ ☐

43. The ergot-derived dopamine receptor agonists include both bromocriptine and lisuride. ☐ ☐

44. Mescaline is an antagonist of phencyclidine. ☐ ☐

45. Permeability of the cell membrane to a drug is proportional to the drug's partition coefficient. ☐ ☐

46. Unlike olanzapine and clozapine, ziprasidone is not metabolised by CYP1A2. ☐ ☐

47. Naloxone can block analgesia induced either by electrical stimulation or acupuncture. ☐ ☐

48. Buprenorphine has a shorter duration of action than morphine. ☐ ☐

49. Respiratory panic-inducing substances include carbon dioxide. ☐ ☐

50. The Chinese have a low risk of developing neuroleptic induced tardive dyskinesia. ☐ ☐

Paper 32

1. **Randomized controlled trials have good external but poor internal validity.**
Ans. **False.** The opposite is true.

2. **Both 5-hydroxytryptamine and substance P are involved in co-transmission in brainstem and spinal cord.**
Ans. **True.**

3. **Unlike type B adverse drug reactions, type A reactions are unpredictable.**
Ans. **False.** The opposite is true.

4. **Diazepam is the treatment of choice for prolonged febrile convulsions.**
Ans. **True.**

5. **The serotonin 2C receptor (HTR2C) gene is located on the long arm of the X chromosome at Xq24.**
Ans. **True.**

6. **Bioavailability of an intravenously administered drug equals unity.**
Ans. **True.**

7. **Cannabinoids produce dose-related increase of intra-ocular pressure.**
Ans. **False.** They produce a dose-related reduction.

8. **Prophylactic folic acid reduces the incidence of neural tube defects due to valproate or carbamazepine.**
Ans. **True.**

9. **The binding of drugs to plasma proteins is irreversible.**
Ans. **False.** It is reversible.

10. **Tricyclic antidepressant drugs have Class Ia antiarrhythmic properties.**
Ans. **True.**

11. **The association between hypothyroidism and the development of rapid cycling course in patients with bipolar I disorder has been shown as independent of the effects of lithium.**
Ans. **True.**

12. **Serotonin antagonists antagonize the effects of hallucinogens.**
Ans. **True.**

13. **SSRIs can cause reversible galactorrhea.**
Ans. **True.** This is due to increased prolactin levels.

14. **Relapse rates after ECT are much higher than those after stopping antidepressants.**
A **False.** They are similar in both scenarios.

15. **The dose of amisulpride should be reduced if the patient's creatinine clearance is low.**
Ans. **True.**

16. **The plasma concentration of diazepam for anxiolytic action is more than that for its anticonvulsant action.**
Ans. **False.**

17. **Recognized side-effects of clonidine include depression.**
Ans. **True.**

18. **Prophylactic treatment of major depressive disorder with antidepressants is effective in reducing the severity but not the number of recurrences.**
Ans. **False.** It is effective in reducing both.

19. **Dopamine receptor antagonists increase the reinforcing effects of amphetamine and cocaine.**
Ans. **False.** They decrease it.

20. **Tetrahydrocannabinol increases slow-wave sleep and reduces REM sleep.**
Ans. **True.**

21. **Chronic alcohol use decreases hepatic metabolism of coadministered drugs.**
Ans. **False.** It increases this.

22. **Quetiapine restores prepulse inhibition of acoustic startle response in apomorphine treated rats.**
Ans. **True.**

23. **Gabapentin is effective for the treatment of neuropathic pain.**
Ans. **True.**

24. **Synergistic interactions between two drugs prescribed together produce a greater effect than the sum of their individual effects.**
Ans. **True.**

25. **A more addictive drug should not be used for detoxification of a patient from a less addictive one.**
Ans. **True.**

26. **Alcohol reduces natural killer cell activity and suppresses B- and T-cell immunity.**
Ans. **True.**

27. **In vitro $5\text{-HT}_{2A}/D_2$ receptor affinity ratio of ziprasidone is lower than that of most other antipsychotic drugs.**
Ans. **False.** Higher.

28. **Noradrenaline is a physiological antagonist for acetylcholine.**
Ans. **True.**

29. **Common side effects of pseudoephedrine include hallucinations.**
Ans. **False.** Hallucinations are rare with this drug.

30. **Patients with cyclothymic disorder are more likely to develop antidepressant-induced hypomania.**
Ans. **True.**

31. **Drug induced tremors are rarely resting tremors.**
Ans. **True.**

32. **Both the dissociation constant of the drug and the pH of its solution determine the extent to which a drug is ionised.**
Ans. **True.**

33. **Predictors of good antimanic response to lithium include substance misuse.**
Ans. **False.** This is a predictor of poor response.

34. **Examples of two neurotransmitters involved together in cotransmission include GABA and glycine in the cerebellum.**
Ans. **True.**

35. **Inhibition caused by drugs occurs slower than enzyme induction.**
Ans. **False.** The opposite is true.

36. **Alcohol is one of the commonest causes of atrial fibrillation.**
Ans. **True.**

37. **$5HT_1$ agonists are effective in the treatment of acute migraine attacks.**
Ans. **True.**

38. Pharmaceutical interactions between two drugs occur during their metabolism.
Ans. **False.** They occur outside the body e.g. in syringe.

39. Buspirone has been associated with extrapyramidal side-effects.
Ans. **True.**

40. Randomized controlled trials of a drug are more generalizable than pragmatic trials.
Ans. **False.** The opposite is true.

41. Adenylyl cyclase and phospholipase C are regulated by G proteins.
Ans. **True.**

42. The CNS depressant actions of the benzodiazepines and alcohol are additive.
Ans. **True.**

43. The ergot-derived dopamine receptor agonists include both bromocriptine and lisuride.
Ans. **True.**

44. Mescaline is an antagonist of phencyclidine.
Ans. **False.** Both are hallucinogens.

45. Permeability of the cell membrane to a drug is proportional to the drug's partition coefficient.
Ans. **True.**

46. Unlike olanzapine and clozapine, ziprasidone is not metabolised by CYP1A2.
Ans. **True.**

47. Naloxone can block analgesia induced either by electrical stimulation or acupuncture.
Ans. **True.**

48. Buprenorphine has a shorter duration of action than morphine.
Ans. **False.** It is longer.

49. Respiratory panic-inducing substances include carbon dioxide.
Ans. **True.**

50. The Chinese have a low risk of developing neuroleptic induced tardive dyskinesia.
Ans. **True.**

Paper 33

	True	False
1. Inhibition of COMT is the main mechanism of action of tranylcypromine.	☐	☐
2. Dopamine–β-hydroxylase uses ascorbic acid as a cofactor in forming noradrenaline from dopamine.	☐	☐
3. Caffeine antagonizes the effects of alcohol.	☐	☐
4. Cyproheptadine is an antihistamine with serotonin-antagonist and calcium channel blocking properties.	☐	☐
5. Lofexidine is more hypotensive than clonidine in the treatment of opioid withdrawal.	☐	☐
6. Antidepressant drugs do not reduce the risk of new depressive episodes.	☐	☐
7. Neurotransmitters are considered as primary messengers.	☐	☐
8. Potency of a drug is represented on the X axis of the dose-response curve.	☐	☐
9. Clozapine's ability to restore prepulse inhibition of the acoustic startle response in apomorphine-treated rats is correlated with its clinical potency as an antipsychotic.	☐	☐
10. κ-opioid receptor agonists are less likely to cause hallucinations than are other opioid agonist drugs.	☐	☐
11. Acetylcholinesterase inhibitors can cause dose-related cholinergic effects.	☐	☐
12. More than half of the patients with cyclothymic disorder are likely to respond to lithium treatment.	☐	☐
13. Biotransformation of a drug always leads to its inactivation.	☐	☐
14. Cocaine inhibits the activity of the dopamine transporter.	☐	☐
15. Clomipramine is contraindicated in pregnancy.	☐	☐
16. Overestimation of the beneficial effects of a drug which leads to publication bias can be identified by funnel plot analysis.	☐	☐
17. Morphine withdrawal symptoms can be reversed by κ (kappa) – opioid receptor agonists.	☐	☐
18. Bupropion is contra-indicated in patients with a history of seizures.	☐	☐
19. Diazepam should not be added to a heparin infusion.	☐	☐
20. Fatal toxicity index of a drug is calculated based on the number of deaths per million prescriptions of the drug.	☐	☐
21. Inheritance of the acetylator status of an individual is an autosomal dominant trait.	☐	☐
22. Pentazocine belongs to the chemical class of benzomorphans.	☐	☐
23. Early response to lithium strongly predicts long-term response to lithium.	☐	☐
24. Propranolol may be useful in treating both essential tremor and tremors associated with thyrotoxicosis.	☐	☐

25. Flumazenil is a GABA$_B$ receptor antagonist with anti-panic properties. ☐ ☐

26. Sleep deprivation has been shown to accelerate the response to antidepressants. ☐ ☐

27. Milnacipran, an SNRI, does not show interactions with cytochrome P450 system. ☐ ☐

28. Pre-treatment plasma GABA levels correlate with the response to lithium. ☐ ☐

29. Clobazam shows anticonvulsant action without producing sedation. ☐ ☐

30. Examples of two neurotransmitters involved together in co-transmission include GABA and 5-HT in the raphae nuclei. ☐ ☐

31. Recognised side-effects of amantadine include hallucinations. ☐ ☐

32. Yohimbine has been shown to be effective in treatment of both idiopathic and medication induced male erectile dysfunction. ☐ ☐

33. Scopolamine is a tricyclic antidepressant. ☐ ☐

34. Dopamine–β–hydroxylase is used as a marker of noradrenergic neuronal activity. ☐ ☐

35. Therapeutic doses of lithium carbonate can worsen psoriasis. ☐ ☐

36. Depakote may give a false positive urine test for ketones. ☐ ☐

37. Both ziprasidone and quetiapine show linear pharmacokinetics. ☐ ☐

38. Lithium has been associated with increased postictal delirium and prolonged seizure activity following ECT. ☐ ☐

39. Renal clearance of a drug is directly proportional to its protein binding. ☐ ☐

40. Serotonergic discontinuation syndrome due to paroxetine withdrawal is more severe than due to fluoxetine withdrawal. ☐ ☐

41. Symptoms of overdose with racemic cipramil include prolonged QT interval. ☐ ☐

42. Zolpidem and zopiclone act primarily on BZ$_3$ receptors. ☐ ☐

43. In treatment of narcolepsy, tolerance does not develop with modafinil. ☐ ☐

44. Antimuscarinic drugs are not as effective as dopaminergic drugs in treatment of idiopathic Parkinson's disease. ☐ ☐

45. Folate deficiency has been associated with dementia but not with depression. ☐ ☐

46. Some cytochrome P450 isoenzymes are not present in some individuals. ☐ ☐

47. Cannabinoids have been shown to produce antinociception. ☐ ☐

48. Coadministration of clozapine and valproate semisodium is contraindicated. ☐ ☐

49. Impairment of the registration and subsequent recall of events has been associated with short-acting benzodiazepines. ☐ ☐

50. Selegeline has shown efficacy in the treatment of narcolepsy. ☐ ☐

Paper 33

1. **Inhibition of COMT is the main mechanism of action of tranylcypromine.**
Ans. **False.** Inhibition of MAO it its main mechamism.

2. **Dopamine–β-hydroxylase uses ascorbic acid as a cofactor in forming noradrenaline from dopamine.**
Ans. **True.**

3. **Caffeine antagonizes the effects of alcohol.**
Ans. **False.**

4. **Cyproheptadine is an antihistamine with serotonin-antagonist and calcium channel blocking properties.**
Ans. **True.**

5. **Lofexidine is more hypotensive than clonidine in the treatment of opioid withdrawal.**
Ans. **False.** It is less hypotensive.

6. **Antidepressant drugs do not reduce the risk of new depressive episodes.**
Ans. **False.**

7. **Neurotransmitters are considered as primary messengers.**
Ans. **True.**

8. **Potency of a drug is represented on the X axis of the dose-response curve.**
Ans. **True.**

9. **Clozapine's ability to restore prepulse inhibition of the acoustic startle response in apomorphine-treated rats is correlated with its clinical potency as an antipsychotic.**
Ans. **True.**

10. **κ-opioid receptor agonists are less likely to cause hallucinations than are other opioid agonist drugs.**
Ans. **False.** They are more likely to cause hallucinations.

11. **Acetylcholinesterase inhibitors can cause dose-related cholinergic effects.**
Ans. **True.**

12. **More than half of the patients with cyclothymic disorder are likely to respond to lithium treatment.**
Ans. **True.**

13. **Biotransformation of a drug always leads to its inactivation.**
Ans. **False.**

14. **Cocaine inhibits the activity of the dopamine transporter.**
Ans. **True.**

15. **Clomipramine is contraindicated in pregnancy.**
Ans. **False.**

16. **Overestimation of the beneficial effects of a drug which leads to publication bias can be identified by funnel plot analysis.**
Ans. **True.**

17. **Morphine withdrawal symptoms can be reversed by κ (kappa) – opioid receptor agonists.**
Ans. **False.** They can be reversed by μ–opioid receptor agonists.

18. Bupropion is contra-indicated in patients with a history of seizures.
Ans. True.

19. Diazepam should not be added to a heparin infusion.
Ans. True. It forms a precipitate.

20. Fatal toxicity index of a drug is calculated based on the number of deaths per million prescriptions of the drug.
Ans. True.

21. Inheritance of the acetylator status of an individual is an autosomal dominant trait.
Ans. False. It is autosomal recessive.

22. Pentazocine belongs to the chemical class of benzomorphans.
Ans. True.

23. Early response to lithium strongly predicts long-term response to lithium.
Ans. True.

24. Propranolol may be useful in treating both essential tremor and tremors associated with thyrotoxicosis.
Ans. True.

25. Flumazenil is a $GABA_B$ receptor antagonist with anti-panic properties.
Ans. False. It is panic-inducing.

26. Sleep deprivation has been shown to accelerate the response to antidepressants.
Ans. True.

27. Milnacipran, an SNRI, does not show interactions with cytochrome P450 system.
Ans. True.

28. Pre-treatment plasma GABA levels correlate with the response to lithium.
Ans. False.

29. Clobazam shows anticonvulsant action without producing sedation.
Ans. True.

30. Examples of two neurotransmitters involved together in co-transmission include GABA and 5-HT in the raphae nuclei.
Ans. True.

31. Recognised side-effects of amantadine include hallucinations.
Ans. True.

32. Yohimbine has been shown to be effective in treatment of both idiopathic and medication induced male erectile dysfunction.
Ans. True.

33. Scopolamine is a tricyclic antidepressant.
Ans. False. It is a muscarinic antagonist.

34. Dopamine−β−hydroxylase is used as a marker of noradrenergic neuronal activity.
Ans. True.

35. Therapeutic doses of lithium carbonate can worsen psoriasis.
Ans. True.

36. Depakote may give a false positive urine test for ketones.
Ans. True.

37. Both ziprasidone and quetiapine show linear pharmacokinetics.

Ans. True.

38. Lithium has been associated with increased postictal delirium and prolonged seizure activity following ECT.

Ans. True.

39. Renal clearance of a drug is directly proportional to its protein binding.

Ans. False. They are inversely proportional.

40. Serotonergic discontinuation syndrome due to paroxetine withdrawal is more severe than due to fluoxetine withdrawal.

Ans. True.

41. Symptoms of overdose with racemic cipramil include prolonged QT interval.

Ans. True.

42. Zolpidem and zopiclone act primarily on BZ_3 receptors.

Ans. False. They act on BZ1 receptors.

43. In treatment of narcolepsy, tolerance does not develop with modafinil.

Ans. True.

44. Antimuscarinic drugs are not as effective as dopaminergic drugs in treatment of idiopathic Parkinson's disease.

Ans. True.

45. Folate deficiency has been associated with dementia but not with depression.

Ans. False. It is associated with both.

46. Some cytochrome P450 isoenzymes are not present in some individuals.

Ans. True.

47. Cannabinoids have been shown to produce antinociception.

Ans. True.

48. Coadministration of clozapine and valproate semisodium is contraindicated.

Ans. False.

49. Impairment of the registration and subsequent recall of events has been associated with short-acting benzodiazepines.

Ans. True.

50. Selegeline has shown efficacy in the treatment of narcolepsy.

Ans. True.

Paper 34

Questions

1. Doses of fosphenytoin should be expressed as phenytoin sodium equivalent. ☐ ☐

2. β-adrenergic receptor antagonists have not shown efficacy in treatment of panic disorder. ☐ ☐

3. Patients who are on irreversible monoamine oxidase inhibitors should avoid fresh herring in their diet. ☐ ☐

4. Efficacy of a drug is represented on the Y axis of the dose-response curve. ☐ ☐

5. Lithium carbonate is a stronger proconvulsant than chlorpromazine. ☐ ☐

6. Brain concentrations of hypocretin-1 and hypocretin-2 have been shown to be reduced in patients with narcolepsy. ☐ ☐

7. Cannabis increases production of α – and β – interferon and the cytolytic activity of macrophages. ☐ ☐

8. In the treatment of bipolar disorders, addition of a psychotherapeutic intervention has been associated with improved compliance with medication. ☐ ☐

9. Diplopia is a recognized side effect of lithium in therapeutic doses. ☐ ☐

10. Cataplexy has been shown to respond to treatment with SSRIs. ☐ ☐

11. Tricyclic antidepressant drugs can block dopamine reuptake in vitro. ☐ ☐

12. Chronic antidepressant treatment has been shown to increase the expression of cAMP response element binding protein (CREB). ☐ ☐

13. Ketamine is a non-competitive antagonist at NMDA receptors. ☐ ☐

14. Metabolism of lithium carbonate includes oxidation followed by conjugation. ☐ ☐

15. Both in vivo and in vitro studies have shown that Δ^9–tetrahydrocannabinol impairs cell-mediated immunity and humoral immunity. ☐ ☐

16. Recognized side effects of valproate semisodium include reversible Fanconi's syndrome. ☐ ☐

17. Steady-state plasma levels of escitalopram are achieved in 48 hours. ☐ ☐

18. Both $5HT_3$ and D_2 receptor antagonists show antiemetic properties. ☐ ☐

19. Decreased ^3H imipramine binding has been shown to normalize with antidepressant treatment. ☐ ☐

20. Muscarinic receptors use G proteins for signal transduction and are metabotropic. ☐ ☐

21. Entacapone provides antiparkinsonian benefit only when used as an adjunt to levodopa. ☐ ☐

22. Sexual functioning side-effects associated with paroxetine are less than that of other SSRIs. ☐ ☐

23. Measuring patient attitude to antipsychotic treatment with self-report instrument predicts adherence 1 year later. ☐ ☐

24. The behavioural and cognitive effects of stimulant medication are not confined to patients with ADHD. ☐ ☐

25. Tertiary amine antidepressants are more selective for the serotonin transporter than the norepinephrine transporter. ☐ ☐

26. Clozapine has been shown to improve P50 suppression (a measure of sensory gating) in patients with schizophrenia. ☐ ☐

27. The Simpson Agnus Scale measures the severity of obsessions and compulsions. ☐ ☐

28. Pleurothotonus has been associated with neuroleptic treatment. ☐ ☐

29. Response to treatment with a drug does not change over the time course of the illness. ☐ ☐

30. Metabolism of alcohol follows zero-order kinetics. ☐ ☐

31. Benzodiazepines do not bind to $GABA_A$ receptors. ☐ ☐

32. Both serotonin and norepinephrine suppress REM sleep. ☐ ☐

33. Paroxetine shows both noradrenergic reuptake inhibition and mild cholinergic receptor blockade. ☐ ☐

34. Partial dopamine receptor agonists show relative intrinsic activity higher than dopamine. ☐ ☐

35. Studies have shown an effect size of 0.8 – 1.2 for stimulant drugs in the treatment of ADHD. ☐ ☐

36. Activation of the postsynaptic receptor always results in membrane depolarisation. ☐ ☐

37. An ideal hypnotic drug should have active metabolites. ☐ ☐

38. The spontaneously hypertensive rat has been used as an animal model of ADHD. ☐ ☐

39. Nicotinic receptors are ionotropic and use ligand-gated ion channels for signal transduction. ☐ ☐

40. The dose response ceiling of a drug is lower for obsessive-compulsive disorder than for panic disorder. ☐ ☐

41. Correlation has been reported between the development of tardive dyskinesia and the DRD3 Ser9Gly polymorphism. ☐ ☐

42. Numbers needed to treat (NNT) with Rivastigmine is 7 , Donepezil is 4 and Galantamine is 3. ☐ ☐

43. Mixed affective state predicts poor response to lithium. ☐ ☐

44. Paliperidone is not bound to cholinergic receptors. ☐ ☐

45. NMDA receptor antagonists may improve psychotic symptoms. ☐ ☐

46. Metoclopramide can cause tardive dyskinesia. ☐ ☐

47. Carbidopa, a peripheral inhibitor of L-DOPA decarboxylase , is used along with L-Dopa in treatment with idiopathic Parkinson's disese. ☐ ☐

48. **Drug induced acute dystonic reactions are more common in older adults than in younger adults.** ☐ ☐

49. **Clozapine-induced seizures are treated with carbamazepine.** ☐ ☐

50. **Vilazodone binds with high affinity to the serotonin reuptake site, but not to the norepinephrine reuptake site.** ☐ ☐

Paper 34

Answers with explanations

1. Doses of fosphenytoin should be expressed as phenytoin sodium equivalent.
Ans. True.

2. β-adrenergic receptor antagonists have not shown efficacy in treatment of panic disorder.
Ans. True.

3. Patients who are on irreversible monoamine oxidase inhibitors should avoid fresh herring in their diet.
Ans. False. They should avoid pickled herring.

4. Efficacy of a drug is represented on the Y axis of the dose-response curve.
Ans. True.

5. Lithium carbonate is a stronger proconvulsant than chlorpromazine.
Ans. False.

6. Brain concentrations of hypocretin-1 and hypocretin-2 have been shown to be reduced in patients with narcolepsy.
Ans. True.

7. Cannabis increases production of α – and β – interferon and the cytolytic activity of macrophages.
Ans. False. It suppresses these.

8. In the treatment of bipolar disorders, addition of a psychotherapeutic intervention has been associated with improved compliance with medication.
Ans. True.

9. Diplopia is a recognized side effect of lithium in therapeutic doses.
Ans. False. This occurs at toxic doses.

10. Cataplexy has been shown to respond to treatment with SSRIs.
Ans. True.

11. Tricyclic antidepressant drugs can block dopamine reuptake in vitro.
Ans. True.

12. Chronic antidepressant treatment has been shown to increase the expression of cAMP response element binding protein (CREB).
Ans. True.

13. Ketamine is a non-competitive antagonist at NMDA receptors.
Ans. True.

14. Metabolism of lithium carbonate includes oxidation followed by conjugation.
Ans. False. Lithium carbonate is not metabolized.

15. Both in vivo and in vitro studies have shown that Δ^9–tetrahydrocannabinol impairs cell-mediated immunity and humoral immunity.
Ans. True.

16. Recognized side effects of valproate semisodium include reversible Fanconi's syndrome.
Ans. True.

17. Steady-state plasma levels of escitalopram are achieved in 48 hours.
Ans. False. This is achieved after one week.

18. Both $5HT_3$ and D_2 receptor antagonists show antiemetic properties.
Ans. True.

19. Decreased ^{3}H imipramine binding has been shown to normalize with antidepressant treatment.
Ans. True.

20. Muscarinic receptors use G proteins for signal transduction and are metabotropic.
Ans. True.

21. Entacapone provides antiparkinsonian benefit only when used as an adjunt to levodopa.
Ans. True.

22. Sexual functioning side-effects associated with paroxetine are less than that of other SSRIs.
Ans. False. More than that of other SSRIs.

23. Measuring patient attitude to antipsychotic treatment with self-report instrument predicts adherence 1 year later.
Ans. True.

24. The behavioural and cognitive effects of stimulant medication are not confined to patients with ADHD.
Ans. True. They are also seen in unaffected children.

25. Tertiary amine antidepressants are more selective for the serotonin transporter than the norepinephrine transporter.
Ans. True.

26. Clozapine has been shown to improve P50 suppression (a measure of sensory gating) in patients with schizophrenia.
Ans. True.

27. The Simpson Agnus Scale measures the severity of obsessions and compulsions.
Ans. False. It meaures antipsychotic induced Parkinsonian side effects.

28. Pleurothotonus has been associated with neuroleptic treatment.
Ans. True. It is known as pisa syndrome.

29. Response to treatment with a drug does not change over the time course of the illness.
Ans. False.

30. Metabolism of alcohol follows zero-order kinetics.
Ans. True.

31. Benzodiazepines do not bind to GABA$_A$ receptors.
Ans. True.

32. Both serotonin and norepinephrine suppress REM sleep.
Ans. True.

33. Paroxetine shows both noradrenergic reuptake inhibition and mild cholinergic receptor blockade.
Ans. True.

34. Partial dopamine receptor agonists show relative intrinsic activity higher than dopamine.
Ans. False. The opposite is true.

35. Studies have shown an effect size of 0.8 – 1.2 for stimulant drugs in the treatment of ADHD.
Ans. True.

36. Activation of the postsynaptic receptor always results in membrane depolarisation.
Ans. False. It results in hyperpolarisation.

37. An ideal hypnotic drug should have active metabolites.
Ans. False.

38. The spontaneously hypertensive rat has been used as an animal model of ADHD.

Ans. True.

39. Nicotinic receptors are ionotropic and use ligand-gated ion channels for signal transduction.

Ans. True.

40. The dose response ceiling of a drug is lower for obsessive-compulsive disorder than for panic disorder.

Ans. False.

41. Correlation has been reported between the development of tardive dyskinesia and the DRD3 Ser9Gly polymorphism.

Ans. True.

42. Numbers needed to treat (NNT) with Rivastigmine is 7 , Donepezil is 4 and Galantamine is 3.

Ans. True.

43. Mixed affective state predicts poor response to lithium.

Ans. True.

44. Paliperidone is not bound to cholinergic receptors.

Ans. True.

45. NMDA receptor antagonists may improve psychotic symptoms.

Ans. False. They may induce psychotic symptoms.

46. Metoclopramide can cause tardive dyskinesia.

Ans. True.

47. Carbidopa, a peripheral inhibitor of L-DOPA decarboxylase , is used along with L-Dopa in treatment with idiopathic Parkinson's disese.

Ans. True.

48. Drug induced acute dystonic reactions are more common in older adults than in younger adults.

Ans. False. Commoner in younger adults.

49. Clozapine-induced seizures are treated with carbamazepine.

Ans. False. They are treated with valproate.

50. Vilazodone binds with high affinity to the serotonin reuptake site, but not to the norepinephrine reuptake site.

Ans. True.

Paper 35

	True	False

1. Hypothalamo-pituitary-adrenal axis abnormalities are not specific to depressive disorder. ☐ ☐

2. It is not recommended that the dosage of an SSRI in increased until its steady state is reached. ☐ ☐

3. Effectiveness of some antiepileptic drugs can be assessed by measurement of GABA in cerebral cortex by proton magnetic resonance spectroscopy. ☐ ☐

4. Muscarinic antagonists are known to enhance REM sleep. ☐ ☐

5. Positive and negative syndrome scale (PANSS) can be used to evaluate response to treatment with antipsychotic drugs. ☐ ☐

6. GABA agonists enhance the binding of benzodiazepines to their receptors. ☐ ☐

7. Doses of a drug given at longer intervals than the half-life of the drug lead to small fluctuations in plasma concentration. ☐ ☐

8. Both sodium valproate and carbamazapine are folic acid antagonists. ☐ ☐

9. Glucuronidation is well preserved in the elderly. ☐ ☐

10. Escitalopram has been shown to be the least selective of all SSRIs. ☐ ☐

11. The dim light melatonin onset (DLMO) can be used as a marker for circadian phase position. ☐ ☐

12. Response to treatment with a psychotropic drug gives a definite guide to construct validity of the disorder. ☐ ☐

13. Both D_1 and D_4 receptors inhibit cAMP. ☐ ☐

14. Dialysis is of no use for the treatment of benzodiazepine overdose. ☐ ☐

15. CYP2D6 activity is not decreased in the elderly. ☐ ☐

16. Amitriptyline was the first drug in the history of psychiatry to act specifically against depression. ☐ ☐

17. Gamma hydroxyl butyrate has hallucinogenic and euphoric effects. ☐ ☐

18. Catechol O-methyltransferase (COMT) inhibitors prolong the elimination half-life of levodopa in treatment of Parkinson's disease. ☐ ☐

19. Open clinical trials are used in the formal evaluation of efficacy of a drug in phase III stage. ☐ ☐

20. A drug with a high volume of distribution (Vd) has low affinity for tissues outside body water. ☐ ☐

21. Discontinuation of normal therapeutic doses of benzodiazepines can produce a withdrawal syndrome. ☐ ☐

22. Anticholinergic drugs delay the absorption of paracetamol. ☐ ☐

23. Benzodiazepine use in the UK has been reported to be more common in men than in women. ☐ ☐

24. Urinary alkalizers prolong pharmacological effects of amphetamine.   ☐   ☐

25. Both carbamazepine and phenytoin attenuate the kindling rate.   ☐   ☐

26. Clonidine stimulates presynaptic α_2 receptors at low doses and postsynaptic α_2 receptors at high doses.   ☐   ☐

27. Cannabinoid (CB_1) agonists inhibit GABA inhibition of dopamine in the ventral tegmental area.   ☐   ☐

28. Acetazolamide reduces elimination of lithium.   ☐   ☐

29. R-citalopram has an inhibitory effect on the effects of escitalopram.   ☐   ☐

30. Muscarinic antagonists are known to impair memory and learning.   ☐   ☐

31. Flunitrazepam causes disinhibition and anterograde amnesia for events that occur under the influence of the drug.   ☐   ☐

32. Dissociative disorders are less likely to show placebo response than dysthymic disorders.   ☐   ☐

33. Both cyclic AMP and inositol trisphosphate activate protein kinases which in turn regulate various cellular functions.   ☐   ☐

34. Consumption of garlic can lead to inhibition of CYP2E1.   ☐   ☐

35. The M_2 and M_4 muscarinic receptors are presynaptic inhibitory autoreceptors that inhibit the release of acetylcholine.   ☐   ☐

36. Galantamine potentiates the action of acetylcholine at nicotinic receptors.   ☐   ☐

37. Melatonin production is reduced by β-blockers but increased by tricyclic antidepressants.   ☐   ☐

38. Sertraline shows moderate dopamine reuptake inhibiting properties.   ☐   ☐

39. Partial agonists at the benzodiazepine receptor are more potent than full agonists.   ☐   ☐

40. A drug achieves its equilibrium in the body during its elimination phase.   ☐   ☐

41. Response to lithium in the treatment of bipolar disorder has been associated with the phospholipase Cy-1 gene.   ☐   ☐

42. Time taken to replace stores of MAO after its irreversible blockade by MAOI is more important than its half-life.   ☐   ☐

43. Osmotic diuretics increase the plasma concentration of lithium.   ☐   ☐

44. Secondary amine antidepressants are more selective for the norepinephrine transporter than the serotonin transporter.   ☐   ☐

45. Long-term use of non-steroidal anti-inflammatory drugs has been associated with increased risk of Alzheimer's disease.   ☐   ☐

46. The oral bioavailability of drugs that are substrates of CYP3A4 is decreased if grapefruit juice is consumed simultaneously.   ☐   ☐

47. Recognised side effects of zolpidem include diplopia.   ☐   ☐

48. Cranberry juice increases excretion of phencyclidine.

49. Benserazide is an amino-acid decarboxylase inhibitor which reduces the bioavailability of levodopa.

50. Stimulant drugs reduce orbitofrontal cerebral activity.

1. **Hypothalamo-pituitary-adrenal axis abnormalities are not specific to depressive disorder.**
Ans. **True.**

2. **It is not recommended that the dosage of an SSRI in increased until its steady state is reached.**
Ans. **True.**

3. **Effectiveness of some antiepileptic drugs can be assessed by measurement of GABA in cerebral cortex by proton magnetic resonance spectroscopy.**
Ans. **True.**

4. **Muscarinic antagonists are known to enhance REM sleep.**
Ans. **False.** They suppress REM sleep.

5. **Positive and negative syndrome scale (PANSS) can be used to evaluate response to treatment with antipsychotic drugs.**
Ans. **True.**

6. **GABA agonists enhance the binding of benzodiazepines to their receptors.**
Ans. **True.**

7. **Doses of a drug given at longer intervals than the half-life of the drug lead to small fluctuations in plasma concentration.**
Ans. **False.** This leads to large fluctuations in plasma concentration.

8. **Both sodium valproate and carbamazapine are folic acid antagonists.**
Ans. **True.**

9. **Glucuronidation is well preserved in the elderly.**
Ans. **True.**

10. **Escitalopram has been shown to be the least selective of all SSRIs.**
Ans. **False.** It is the most selective.

11. **The dim light melatonin onset (DLMO) can be used as a marker for circadian phase position.**
Ans. **True.**

12. **Response to treatment with a psychotropic drug gives a definite guide to construct validity of the disorder.**
Ans. **False.**

13. **Both D_1 and D_4 receptors inhibit cAMP.**
Ans. **False.** D_1 receptors do not do this.

14. **Dialysis is of no use for the treatment of benzodiazepine overdose.**
Ans. **True.** This is due to their high lipid solubility and large volume of distribution.

15. **CYP2D6 activity is not decreased in the elderly.**
Ans. **True.**

16. **Amitriptyline was the first drug in the history of psychiatry to act specifically against depression.**
Ans. **False.** Imipramine was.

17. **Gamma hydroxyl butyrate has hallucinogenic and euphoric effects.**
Ans. **True.**

18. **Catechol O-methyltransferase (COMT) inhibitors prolong the elimination half-life of levodopa in treatment of Parkinson's disease.**
Ans. **True.**

19. Open clinical trials are used in the formal evaluation of efficacy of a drug in phase III stage.
Ans. **False.** This happens at phase II.

20. A drug with a high volume of distribution (Vd) has low affinity for tissues outside body water.
Ans. **False.** It has high affinity.

21. Discontinuation of normal therapeutic doses of benzodiazepines can produce a withdrawal syndrome.
Ans. **True.**

22. Anticholinergic drugs delay the absorption of paracetamol.
Ans. **True.** By decreasing peristalsis.

23. Benzodiazepine use in the UK has been reported to be more common in men than in women.
Ans. **False.** It is more common in women.

24. Urinary alkalizers prolong pharmacological effects of amphetamine.
Ans. **True.**

25. Both carbamazepine and phenytoin attenuate the kindling rate.
Ans. **False.** Phenytoin does not do this.

26. Clonidine stimulates presynaptic α_2 receptors at low doses and postsynaptic α_2 receptors at high doses.
Ans. **True.**

27. Cannabinoid (CB_1) agonists inhibit GABA inhibition of dopamine in the ventral tegmental area.
Ans. **True.**

28. Acetazolamide reduces elimination of lithium.
Ans. **False.** It accelerates it.

29. R-citalopram has an inhibitory effect on the effects of escitalopram.
Ans. **True.**

30. Muscarinic antagonists are known to impair memory and learning.
Ans. **True.**

31. Flunitrazepam causes disinhibition and anterograde amnesia for events that occur under the influence of the drug.
Ans. **True.**

32. Dissociative disorders are less likely to show placebo response than dysthymic disorders.
Ans. **False.** They are more likely to do this.

33. Both cyclic AMP and inositol trisphosphate activate protein kinases which in turn regulate various cellular functions.
Ans. **True.**

34. Consumption of garlic can lead to inhibition of CYP2E1.
Ans. **True.** By its component diallysulphide.

35. The M_2 and M_4 muscarinic receptors are presynaptic inhibitory autoreceptors that inhibit the release of acetylcholine.
Ans. **True.**

36. Galantamine potentiates the action of acetylcholine at nicotinic receptors.
Ans. **True.**

37. Melatonin production is reduced by β-blockers but increased by tricyclic antidepressants.
Ans. **True.**

38. Sertraline shows moderate dopamine reuptake inhibiting properties.

Ans. True.

39. Partial agonists at the benzodiazepine receptor are more potent than full agonists.

Ans. False. They are less potent.

40. A drug achieves its equilibrium in the body during its elimination phase.

Ans. False. This occurs during distribution phase.

41. Response to lithium in the treatment of bipolar disorder has been associated with the phospholipase Cy-1 gene.

Ans. True.

42. Time taken to replace stores of MAO after its irreversible blockade by MAOI is more important than its half-life.

Ans. True.

43. Osmotic diuretics increase the plasma concentration of lithium.

Ans. False. They reduce this.

44. Secondary amine antidepressants are more selective for the norepinephrine transporter than the serotonin transporter.

Ans. True.

45. Long-term use of non-steroidal anti-inflammatory drugs has been associated with increased risk of Alzheimer's disease.

Ans. False. They are associated with a decreased risk.

46. The oral bioavailability of drugs that are substrates of CYP3A4 is decreased if grapefruit juice is consumed simultaneously.

Ans. False. It is increased.

47. Recognised side effects of zolpidem include diplopia.

Ans. True.

48. Cranberry juice increases excretion of phencyclidine.

Ans. True.

49. Benserazide is an amino-acid decarboxylase inhibitor which reduces the bioavailability of levodopa.

Ans. False. It increases the bioavailability of levodopa.

50. Stimulant drugs reduce orbitofrontal cerebral activity.

Ans. False. They increase this.

Paper 36

		True	False
1.	Clozapine causes an increase in EEG slow wave activity.	☐	☐
2.	Inverse agonists of benzodiazepine receptors have anticonvulsant and anxiolytic actions.	☐	☐
3.	Alcohol and phenytoin are examples of drugs for which clearance is not constant.	☐	☐
4.	Enantiomers of a drug differ in their ability to rotate plane-polarized light.	☐	☐
5.	The ergot-derived dopamine agonists used in treatment of Parkinson's disease are known to cause pleuropulmonary fibrosis.	☐	☐
6.	Obsessive-compulsive disorder is more likely to show placebo response than adjustment disorder.	☐	☐
7.	Valproate is heavily protein bound compared to gabapentin.	☐	☐
8.	GABA-B receptor agonists have antinociceptive properties.	☐	☐
9.	Dopamine antagonists block the apomorphine-induced climbing behaviour in mice.	☐	☐
10.	The dopamine D2 receptor (DRD2) gene is located on chromosome 15.	☐	☐
11.	Selective MAO-B inhibitors do not cause the cheese reaction.	☐	☐
12.	Blood-brain barrier is prominent in the median eminence of the hypothalamus.	☐	☐
13.	Tolerance has been reported to develop to the neurophysiological effects of benzodiazepines.	☐	☐
14.	Gabapentin does not undergo hepatic metabolism.	☐	☐
15.	Haloperidol induces c-fos expression in dorsolateral striatum.	☐	☐
16.	Tests to measure the effects of antipsychotic drugs on cognitive functions in patients with schizophrenia include the Stroop test.	☐	☐
17.	Rate of glucose oxidation in GABAergic neurons can be measured by *in vivo* magnetic resonance spectroscopy.	☐	☐
18.	Stimulant drugs used in ADHD promote stimulus discrimination.	☐	☐
19.	The levorotatory optical isomer of MDMA is more potent than the dextrorotatory isomer.	☐	☐
20.	In the living human brain SPECT measures function, biochemistry and pharmacokinetics of a drug unlike CT.	☐	☐
21.	Progressive worsening of symptoms by repeated administration of stimulants is described as reverse tolerance.	☐	☐
22.	Metabolism of lorazepam involves only the phase II.	☐	☐
23.	In the brain, MAO-B is mostly found extraneuronally, with the exception of serotenergic neurons of the raphe nuclei.	☐	☐
24.	For severe depression antidepressant drug treatment shows similar efficacy to psychological therapies.	☐	☐
25.	Citalopram is a racemic compound, composed of 2 isomers in equal proportions.	☐	☐

26. Clozapine-induced agranulocytosis commonly occurs in the first three months of treatment. ☐ ☐

27. Antagonism of stimulant-induced hyperactivity can be used to detect the efficacy of antidepressant drugs. ☐ ☐

28. Incidences of psychotropic drug metabolic polymorphisms are equal among all populations. ☐ ☐

29. The fetal liver can metabolize drugs. ☐ ☐

30. Aspirin has been shown to improve cognition in vascular dementia. ☐ ☐

31. The Barnes Akathisia Rating Scale includes subjective items and excludes objective items. ☐ ☐

32. The binding affinity of a radioligand to a receptor is directly proportional to its equilibrium dissociation constant (Kd). ☐ ☐

33. Olanzapine has discriminative stimulus properties similar to those of clozapine. ☐ ☐

34. Tachyphylaxis to a single dose of benzodiazepine can be demonstrated on a clockwise hysteresis curve. ☐ ☐

35. Both COMT and MAO inhibitors are used in the treatment of Parkinson's disease. ☐ ☐

36. Symptoms of benzodiazepine withdrawal syndrome include hyposensitivity to stimuli. ☐ ☐

37. During pregnancy, drug absorption is usually decreased and elimination increased. ☐ ☐

38. Baclofen has been shown to blunt both limbic activation and craving in response to cocaine cues. ☐ ☐

39. Continuation treatment with antidepressant drugs beyond 6 months after full remission is recommended in the elderly. ☐ ☐

40. Risk of developing neuroleptic malignant syndrome is low in hot weather. ☐ ☐

41. SSRIs have been shown to be effective in suppressing non paraphilic hypersexuality. ☐ ☐

42. Symptoms of behavioural toxicity due to benzodiazepines include aggression and disinhibition. ☐ ☐

43. Cholinesterase inhibitors are antagonised by antimuscarinic drugs. ☐ ☐

44. The brief psychiatric rating scale includes abnormal motor movements. ☐ ☐

45. The concentration of cannabinoid receptors in cerebellum is very low. ☐ ☐

46. Both receptor sensitivity and receptor numbers are reduced in old age. ☐ ☐

47. Risk of seizures increases with increased doses of clozapine. ☐ ☐

48. Phencyclidine acts as a non competitive NMDA antagonist. ☐ ☐

49. Medroxyprogesterone acetate inhibits the enzyme testosterone reductase. ☐ ☐

50. In animal models of schizophrenia, it has been demonstrated that olanzapine produces catalepsy at doses lower than those required to block the avoidance response. ☐ ☐

Paper 36

1. **Clozapine causes an increase in EEG slow wave activity.**
Ans. True.

2. **Inverse agonists of benzodiazepine receptors have anticonvulsant and anxiolytic actions.**
Ans. False. They are convulsant and anxiogenic.

3. **Alcohol and phenytoin are examples of drugs for which clearance is not constant.**
Ans. True.

4. **Enantiomers of a drug differ in their ability to rotate plane-polarized light.**
Ans. True.

5. **The ergot-derived dopamine agonists used in treatment of Parkinson's disease are known to cause pleuropulmonary fibrosis.**
Ans. True.

6. **Obsessive-compulsive disorder is more likely to show placebo response than adjustment disorder.**
Ans. False. It is less likely to do this.

7. **Valproate is heavily protein bound compared to gabapentin.**
Ans. True.

8. **GABA-B receptor agonists have antinociceptive properties.**
Ans. True.

9. **Dopamine antagonists block the apomorphine-induced climbing behaviour in mice.**
Ans. True.

10. **The dopamine D2 receptor (DRD2) gene is located on chromosome 15.**
Ans. False. Chromosome 11 at 11q23.

11. **Selective MAO-B inhibitors do not cause the cheese reaction.**
Ans. True.

12. **Blood-brain barrier is prominent in the median eminence of the hypothalamus.**
Ans. False. It is absent.

13. **Tolerance has been reported to develop to the neurophysiological effects of benzodiazepines.**
Ans. True. For example, EEG fast wave activity.

14. **Gabapentin does not undergo hepatic metabolism.**
Ans. True.

15. **Haloperidol induces c-fos expression in dorsolateral striatum.**
Ans. True. This is related to extrapyramidal effects.

16. **Tests to measure the effects of antipsychotic drugs on cognitive functions in patients with schizophrenia include the Stroop test.**
Ans. True.

17. **Rate of glucose oxidation in GABAergic neurons can be measured by *in vivo* magnetic resonance spectroscopy.**
Ans. True.

18. **Stimulant drugs used in ADHD promote stimulus discrimination.**
Ans. True.

19. The levorotatory optical isomer of MDMA is more potent than the dextrorotatory isomer.
Ans. **False.** The opposite is true.

20. In the living human brain SPECT measures function, biochemistry and pharmacokinetics of a drug unlike CT.
Ans. **True.**

21. Progressive worsening of symptoms by repeated administration of stimulants is described as reverse tolerance.
Ans. **True.**

22. Metabolism of lorazepam involves only the phase II.
Ans. **True.**

23. In the brain, MAO-B is mostly found extraneuronally, with the exception of serotenergic neurons of the raphe nuclei.
Ans. **True.**

24. For severe depression antidepressant drug treatment shows similar efficacy to psychological therapies.
Ans. **False.** It shows superior efficacy.

25. Citalopram is a racemic compound, composed of 2 isomers in equal proportions.
Ans. **True.**

26. Clozapine-induced agranulocytosis commonly occurs in the first three months of treatment.
Ans. **True.**

27. Antagonism of stimulant-induced hyperactivity can be used to detect the efficacy of antidepressant drugs.
Ans. **False.** It is used for antipsychotic drugs.

28. Incidences of psychotropic drug metabolic polymorphisms are equal among all populations.
Ans. **False.** Differences exist between Caucasians and Asians.

29. The fetal liver can metabolize drugs.
Ans. **True.**

30. Aspirin has been shown to improve cognition in vascular dementia.
Ans. **True.**

31. The Barnes Akathisia Rating Scale includes subjective items and excludes objective items.
Ans. **False.** It includes both subjective and objective items.

32. The binding affinity of a radioligand to a receptor is directly proportional to its equilibrium dissociation constant (Kd).
Ans. **False.** They are inversely proportional.

33. Olanzapine has discriminative stimulus properties similar to those of clozapine.
Ans. **True.**

34. Tachyphylaxis to a single dose of benzodiazepine can be demonstrated on a clockwise hysteresis curve.
Ans. **True.**

35. Both COMT and MAO inhibitors are used in the treatment of Parkinson's disease.
Ans. **True.**

36. Symptoms of benzodiazepine withdrawal syndrome include hyposensitivity to stimuli.
Ans. **False.** It can cause hypersensitivity.

37. During pregnancy, drug absorption is usually decreased and elimination increased.
Ans. **True.**

38. Baclofen has been shown to blunt both limbic activation and craving in response to cocaine cues.
Ans. True.

39. Continuation treatment with antidepressant drugs beyond 6 months after full remission is recommended in the elderly.
Ans. True.

40. Risk of developing neuroleptic malignant syndrome is low in hot weather.
Ans. False. The risk is high in hot weather.

41. SSRIs have been shown to be effective in suppressing non paraphilic hypersexuality.
Ans. True.

42. Symptoms of behavioural toxicity due to benzodiazepines include aggression and disinhibition.
Ans. True.

43. Cholinesterase inhibitors are antagonised by antimuscarinic drugs.
Ans. True.

44. The brief psychiatric rating scale includes abnormal motor movements.
Ans. True.

45. The concentration of cannabinoid receptors in cerebellum is very low.
Ans. False. It is very high.

46. Both receptor sensitivity and receptor numbers are reduced in old age.
Ans. False. Receptor sensitivity increases in old age.

47. Risk of seizures increases with increased doses of clozapine.
Ans. True. The risk is 1% below 300 mg and 4.4% above 600 mg.

48. Phencyclidine acts as a non competitive NMDA antagonist.
Ans. True.

49. Medroxyprogesterone acetate inhibits the enzyme testosterone reductase.
Ans. False. It induces this.

50. In animal models of schizophrenia, it has been demonstrated that olanzapine produces catalepsy at doses lower than those required to block the avoidance response.
Ans. False. This occurs at higher doses.

Paper 37

	True	False

1. **Among cholinesterase inhibitors, donepezil is a piperidine derivative and rivastigmine is a carbamate derivative.**

2. **Cross-tolerance occurs between PCP and LSD.**

3. **Risk of extra pyramidal side effects due to antipsychotic drugs is low in Lewy-body dementia.**

4. **Loss of gag reflex is a recognised side effect of second generation antipsychotic drugs.**

5. **Benzodiazepines do not cause retrograde amnesia.**

6. **Paroxetine decreases plasma concentrations of galantamine.**

7. **NMDA-receptor agonists (L-glutamate) can stimulate PCP receptors.**

8. **Hyponatraemia due to antidepressant drugs is less common in the elderly than in the younger patients.**

9. **Chronic use of chlorpromazine can cause pigmentation of the Descemet's membrane of the cornea.**

10. **Androgen receptor blockade results in a decrease in both deviant and non-deviant sexual fantasies.**

11. **The Simpson-Angus Scale measures bradykinesia-rigidity, tremor and tardive dyskinesia.**

12. **The extent of dopamine transporter blockade by cocaine is directly proportional to its potential to induce a high.**

13. **Delusional depression in the elderly is less resistant to pharmacotherapy than in younger patients.**

14. **Fluphenazine is esterified with decanoic acid and dissolved in sesame oil to form its depot form.**

15. **Signs of antidepressant-induced hypontraemia include seizures.**

16. **Chlorpromazine is contraindicated in a patient with hypertensive crisis induced by co-administration of MAOIs and tyramine-containing foods.**

17. **Lobeline is a partial nicotine receptor agonist from the Indian tobacco plant.**

18. **The addition of tri-iodothyronine (T_3) to antidepressant medication has been associated with increased response rates in younger patients with treatment-resistant depression.**

19. **PET studies of flumazenil binding have shown a reduction in number of benzodiazepine receptors by 20% in patients with panic disorder.**

20. **Serum lithium levels are increased in hypoalbuminaemia.**

21. **Ethanol acts as an NMDA glutamate receptor antagonist.**

22. **Tolerance develops more readily to the sedative effects of benzodiazepines than to their anxiolytic effects.**

	True	False

23. Reversal of NMDA antagonist-induced reduction in the prepulse inhibition of a startle response has been demonstrated with both quetiapine and olanzapine. ☐ ☐

24. K-opioid receptor activation plays a role in opiate reinforcement. ☐ ☐

25. Lithium toxicity may occur in the elderly when plasma levels are within the therapeutic range. ☐ ☐

26. Citalopram is contraindicated in patients with post-stroke depression who are also on warfarin. ☐ ☐

27. Both corticotrophin-releasing factor (CRF) and thyrotrophin-releasing hormone are synthesized in the paraventricular nucleus of the hypothalamus. ☐ ☐

28. Pharmacokinetics of a drug can be studied by measuring the kinetics of [^{11}C] – labelled drugs by using PET. ☐ ☐

29. The onset of antidepressant discontinuation symptoms is independent of the half-life of the antidepressant. ☐ ☐

30. The concentration of lithium inside RBCs is more than in plasma. ☐ ☐

31. Acute poisoning by mercurial compounds presents with an acute cerebellar syndrome. ☐ ☐

32. Somatostatin concentrations have been reported to be elevated in Alzheimer's disease. ☐ ☐

33. Adding reboxetine to an SSRI leads to serotonin syndrome. ☐ ☐

34. Benzodiazepines cause induction of hepatic microsomal enzymes. ☐ ☐

35. Rat paw test has been used to differentiate the atypical antipsychotics from the first generation antipsychotics. ☐ ☐

36. Amphetamine-like psychostimulants inhibit the binding of dopamine to the dopamine transporter. ☐ ☐

37. Lurasidone shows very high affinity for the 5HT7 and 5HT1A receptors and a low affinity for 5HT2C receptors. ☐ ☐

38. Demyelination of corpus callosum is a recognised common complication of chronic alcohol dependence. ☐ ☐

39. Neuroleptic induced adult-onset focal dystonias include blepharaspasm. ☐ ☐

40. SSRIs have been shown to be effective in controlling impulsivity in borderline personality disorder. ☐ ☐

41. CCK$_B$ (Cholecystokinin) receptor antagonists have been reported to be anxiogenic in animal models. ☐ ☐

42. Compared to younger people, the elderly are more sensitive to benzodiazepine withdrawal symptoms and take longer time to come off the drug. ☐ ☐

43. Serotonin is an inhibitor of feeding. ☐ ☐

44. NMDA receptors are lowest in the cortex and hippocampus. ☐ ☐

45. Drugs with anticholinergic actions can precipitate angle closure by dilating the pupil. ☐ ☐

46. **Inhibition of the action of MAO-A and B enzymes by irreversible MAOI drugs reaches maximum in 48 hours.** ☐ ☐

47. **Chemical transmission by peptides is faster than by neurotransmitters.** ☐ ☐

48. **The sedative and anxiolytic effects of ethanol are associated with facilitation of the GABA-A receptor.** ☐ ☐

49. **Lithium inhibits noradrenaline-induced CAMP activity.** ☐ ☐

50. **Mutations at the RYR1 (ryanodine receptor) site are associated with neuroleptic malignant syndrome.** ☐ ☐

Paper 37

1. Among cholinesterase inhibitors, donepezil is a piperidine derivative and rivastigmine is a carbamate derivative.
Ans. True.

2. Cross-tolerance occurs between PCP and LSD.
Ans. True.

3. Risk of extra pyramidal side effects due to antipsychotic drugs is low in Lewy-body dementia.
Ans. False.

4. Loss of gag reflex is a recognised side effect of second generation antipsychotic drugs.
Ans. True.

5. Benzodiazepines do not cause retrograde amnesia.
Ans. True. They cause anterograde amnesia.

6. Paroxetine decreases plasma concentrations of galantamine.
Ans. False. It increases this.

7. NMDA-receptor agonists (L-glutamate) can stimulate PCP receptors.
Ans. True.

8. Hyponatraemia due to antidepressant drugs is less common in the elderly than in the younger patients.
Ans. False. It is more common in the elderly.

9. Chronic use of chlorpromazine can cause pigmentation of the Descemet's membrane of the cornea.
Ans. True.

10. Androgen receptor blockade results in a decrease in both deviant and non-deviant sexual fantasies.
Ans. True.

11. The Simpson-Angus Scale measures bradykinesia-rigidity, tremor and tardive dyskinesia.
Ans. False. It does not measure tardive dyskinesia.

12. The extent of dopamine transporter blockade by cocaine is directly proportional to its potential to induce a high.
Ans. True.

13. Delusional depression in the elderly is less resistant to pharmacotherapy than in younger patients.
Ans. False. It is more resistant in the elderly.

14. Fluphenazine is esterified with decanoic acid and dissolved in sesame oil to form its depot form.
Ans. True.

15. Signs of antidepressant-induced hypontraemia include seizures.
Ans. True.

16. Chlorpromazine is contraindicated in a patient with hypertensive crisis induced by co-administration of MAOIs and tyramine-containing foods.
Ans. False. It can be beneficial as it causes an α-blockade.

17. Lobeline is a partial nicotine receptor agonist from the Indian tobacco plant.
Ans. True.

18. The addition of tri-iodothyronine (T_3) to antidepressant medication has been associated with increased response rates in younger patients with treatment-resistant depression.
Ans. True.

19. **PET studies of flumazenil binding have shown a reduction in number of benzodiazepine receptors by 20% in patients with panic disorder.**
Ans. True.

20. **Serum lithium levels are increased in hypoalbuminaemia.**
Ans. False. Lithium is not bound to serum proteins.

21. **Ethanol acts as an NMDA glutamate receptor antagonist.**
Ans. True.

22. **Tolerance develops more readily to the sedative effects of benzodiazepines than to their anxiolytic effects.**
Ans. True.

23. **Reversal of NMDA antagonist-induced reduction in the prepulse inhibition of a startle response has been demonstrated with both quetiapine and olanzapine.**
Ans. True.

24. **K-opioid receptor activation plays a role in opiate reinforcement.**
Ans. False.

25. **Lithium toxicity may occur in the elderly when plasma levels are within the therapeutic range.**
Ans. True.

26. **Citalopram is contraindicated in patients with post-stroke depression who are also on warfarin.**
Ans. False. It is recommended in such patients.

27. **Both corticotrophin-releasing factor (CRF) and thyrotrophin-releasing hormone are synthesized in the paraventricular nucleus of the hypothalamus.**
Ans. True.

28. **Pharmacokinetics of a drug can be studied by measuring the kinetics of [^{11}C] – labelled drugs by using PET.**
Ans. True.

29. **The onset of antidepressant discontinuation symptoms is independent of the half-life of the antidepressant.**
Ans. False.

30. **The concentration of lithium inside RBCs is more than in plasma.**
Ans. False. It is less.

31. **Acute poisoning by mercurial compounds presents with an acute cerebellar syndrome.**
Ans. True.

32. **Somatostatin concentrations have been reported to be elevated in Alzheimer's disease.**
Ans. False. They are reduced.

33. **Adding reboxetine to an SSRI leads to serotonin syndrome.**
Ans. False. Reboxetine is a NARI.

34. **Benzodiazepines cause induction of hepatic microsomal enzymes.**
Ans. False.

35. **Rat paw test has been used to differentiate the atypical antipsychotics from the first generation antipsychotics.**
Ans. True.

36. **Amphetamine-like psychostimulants inhibit the binding of dopamine to the dopamine transporter.**
Ans. True.

37. **Lurasidone shows very high affinity for the 5HT7 and 5HT1A receptors and a low affinity for 5HT2C receptors.**
Ans. **True.**

38. **Demyelination of corpus callosum is a recognised common complication of chronic alcohol dependence.**
Ans. **False.** It is rare.

39. **Neuroleptic induced adult-onset focal dystonias include blepharaspasm.**
Ans. **True.**

40. **SSRIs have been shown to be effective in controlling impulsivity in borderline personality disorder.**
Ans. **True.**

41. **CCK$_B$ (Cholecystokinin) receptor antagonists have been reported to be anxiogenic in animal models.**
Ans. **False.** They are anxiolytic.

42. **Compared to younger people, the elderly are more sensitive to benzodiazepine withdrawal symptoms and take longer time to come off the drug.**
Ans. **True.**

43. **Serotonin is an inhibitor of feeding.**
Ans. **True.**

44. **NMDA receptors are lowest in the cortex and hippocampus.**
Ans. **False.** They are at their highest here.

45. **Drugs with anticholinergic actions can precipitate angle closure by dilating the pupil.**
Ans. **True.**

46. **Inhibition of the action of MAO-A and B enzymes by irreversible MAOI drugs reaches maximum in 48 hours.**
Ans. **False.** Up to 2 weeks.

47. **Chemical transmission by peptides is faster than by neurotransmitters.**
Ans. **False.** It is slower.

48. **The sedative and anxiolytic effects of ethanol are associated with facilitation of the GABA-A receptor.**
Ans. **True.**

49. **Lithium inhibits noradrenaline-induced CAMP activity.**
Ans. **True.**

50. **Mutations at the RYR1 (ryanodine receptor) site are associated with neuroleptic malignant syndrome.**
Ans. **False.** They are associated with malignant hyperthermia.

Paper 38

	True	False

1. Psychostimulant treatment causes initial worsening of tics in patients with Tourette's syndrome.

2. Prophylactic treatment with lithium in bipolar disorder reduces the frequency of manic episodes but does not reduce the mortality due to the illness.

3. Chronic administration of clozapine does not cause depolarization block in striatal-projecting dopaminergic cells.

4. Drug-induced type β adverse reactions include allergic dermatological reactions to the drug.

5. Concurrent administration of digitalis preparations and a diuretic that causes potassium loss can cause digitalis delirium.

6. Patients with the DRD2 A1 allele treated with antipsychotic medications have been associated with lower risk of hyperprolactinaemia than patients without this allele.

7. The objectives of effective regulatory pharmacovigilance include long term monitoring of drug safety in clinical practice after marketing.

8. Lithium treatment should be avoided if glomerular filtration rate is less than 30 ml per minute.

9. Antidepressant discontinuation symptoms may occur after missed doses if the antidepressant administered has a short half-life.

10. Neuropeptide Y is a potent appetite inhibiting neurotransmitter.

11. Drug induced increase in intraocular pressure is more common in individuals with narrow irido-corneal angles.

12. Benzodiazepine overdose commonly causes hypoactive delirium.

13. Direct–to–consumer advertising of psychotropic drugs by pharmaceutical companies is more common in Europe than in the USA.

14. Metabolism of a drug usually produces metabolites with increasing water solubility and decreasing lipid solubility.

15. Patients with unipolar depression respond better than those with bipolar depression to treatment with lithium.

16. Corticosteroids are known to cause cataracts.

17. The electroencephalogram (EEG) can be used to investigate drug-induced changes in central arousal.

18. Worsening of OCD symptoms in children is a common complication of chronic use of psychostimulant drugs.

19. Deaths in patients on combination treatments with antidepressants and other drugs are more common in drug misusers.

20. In vitro potency of a drug does not necessarily equate with its in vivo efficacy.

21. Liver biopsy in psychotropic drug-induced acute-onset obstructive-type jaundice shows centrilobular cholestasis.

22. Patients with anxiety disorders are less sensitive to the stimulant and anxiogenic effects of caffeine. ☐ ☐

23. Lithium induced myo-inositol reduction is maximum after only 5 days of lithium administration. ☐ ☐

24. The dose-response function in studies of learning and memory is characterised by an inverted U shape. ☐ ☐

25. Lithium induced hypothyroidism is less common in the presence of antithyroid antibodies. ☐ ☐

26. Drug induced anticholinergic effects are grouped under type B adverse reactions. ☐ ☐

27. Features of the fetal alcohol syndrome include optic nerve hypoplasia. ☐ ☐

28. Sensitisation to a drug refers to an increase in activity due to repeated application of the drug. ☐ ☐

29. Defective oxidation of drugs involving CYP2D6 is more common in Asians than in Caucasians. ☐ ☐

30. Psychostimulant drugs display cross sensitization. ☐ ☐

31. Examples of drug induced behavioural teratogenicity include learning disability. ☐ ☐

32. Common psychotropic drug-induced dermatological reactions include exanthematous reactions. ☐ ☐

33. Plasma concentrations of antiparkinsonian drugs are correlated with improvement in psychotic symptoms when treated with neuroleptic drugs. ☐ ☐

34. Antipsychotic drug treatment induces abdominal fat deposition. ☐ ☐

35. A sigmoid dose-response curve of a drug illustrates the dose of the drug required to produce the maximal effect (Emax). ☐ ☐

36. Reported biochemical changes associated with schizophrenia include decreased $GABA_A$ binding sites in cingulate cortex. ☐ ☐

37. The rate of transfer of a drug across the placental barrier is dependent on the concentration gradient between mother and foetus. ☐ ☐

38. Decreased levels of serum aspartate aminotransferase has been associated with treatment with antipsychotic drugs. ☐ ☐

39. Hypothermia is a recognised complication of neuroleptic drugs. ☐ ☐

40. Carbamazepine may lower free thyroid hormone concentration. ☐ ☐

41. It is possible for a patient to have both drug-induced Parkinsonism and Parkinson's disease. ☐ ☐

42. The binding of an antidepressant drug to the 5-HT and NA reuptake sites is most balanced if its NA/5-HT ratio is closest to 1.0. ☐ ☐

43. Antidepressant-induced seizures are more likely to occur in first-born subjects. ☐ ☐

44. Propranolol increases clearance of diazepam. ☐ ☐

45. **Antipsychotic drugs block dopamine agonist-induced behaviours in rats, like climbing, eye blink and locomotor activity.** ☐   ☐

46. **Lithium-induced tremor is more frequent in younger patients than in elderly patients.** ☐   ☐

47. **Pregabalin binds potently to the alpha-2-delta protein in the brain.** ☐   ☐

48. **Duloxetine has shown efficacy in the treatment of stress urinary incontinence in women.** ☐   ☐

49. **Chlorpromazine-related agranulocytosis has been reported to be less common in individuals of Afro-Caribbean ethnic origin.** ☐   ☐

50. **Clozapine induces depolarization blockade in the nigrostriatal (A9) neurons.** ☐   ☐

1. **Psychostimulant treatment causes initial worsening of tics in patients with Tourette's syndrome.**
Ans. **True.**

2. **Prophylactic treatment with lithium in bipolar disorder reduces the frequency of manic episodes but does not reduce the mortality due to the illness.**
Ans. **False.** It reduces mortality.

3. **Chronic administration of clozapine does not cause depolarization block in striatal-projecting dopaminergic cells.**
Ans. **True.**

4. **Drug-induced type β adverse reactions include allergic dermatological reactions to the drug.**
Ans. **True.**

5. **Concurrent administration of digitalis preparations and a diuretic that causes potassium loss can cause digitalis delirium.**
Ans. **True.**

6. **Patients with the DRD2 A1 allele treated with antipsychotic medications have been associated with lower risk of hyperprolactinaemia than patients without this allele.**
Ans. **False.** They have an increased risk.

7. **The objectives of effective regulatory pharmacovigilance include long term monitoring of drug safety in clinical practice after marketing.**
Ans. **True.**

8. **Lithium treatment should be avoided if glomerular filtration rate is less than 30 ml per minute.**
Ans. **True.**

9. **Antidepressant discontinuation symptoms may occur after missed doses if the antidepressant administered has a short half-life.**
Ans. **True.**

10. **Neuropeptide Y is a potent appetite inhibiting neurotransmitter.**
Ans. **False.** It stimulates the appetite.

11. **Drug induced increase in intraocular pressure is more common in individuals with narrow irido-corneal angles.**
Ans. **True.**

12. **Benzodiazepine overdose commonly causes hypoactive delirium.**
Ans. **True.**

13. **Direct–to–consumer advertising of psychotropic drugs by pharmaceutical companies is more common in Europe than in the USA.**
Ans. **False.**

14. **Metabolism of a drug usually produces metabolites with increasing water solubility and decreasing lipid solubility.**
Ans. **True.**

15. **Patients with unipolar depression respond better than those with bipolar depression to treatment with lithium.**
Ans. **False.** Patients with bipolar depression respond better.

16. **Corticosteroids are known to cause cataracts.**
Ans. **True.**

17. The electroencephalogram (EEG) can be used to investigate drug-induced changes in central arousal.
Ans. True.

18. Worsening of OCD symptoms in children is a common complication of chronic use of psychostimulant drugs.
Ans. False. It is rare.

19. Deaths in patients on combination treatments with antidepressants and other drugs are more common in drug misusers.
Ans. True.

20. In vitro potency of a drug does not necessarily equate with its in vivo efficacy.
Ans. True.

21. Liver biopsy in psychotropic drug-induced acute-onset obstructive-type jaundice shows centrilobular cholestasis.
Ans. True.

22. Patients with anxiety disorders are less sensitive to the stimulant and anxiogenic effects of caffeine.
Ans. False. These patients are more sensitive.

23. Lithium induced myo-inositol reduction is maximum after only 5 days of lithium administration.
Ans. True.

24. The dose-response function in studies of learning and memory is characterised by an inverted U shape.
Ans. True.

25. Lithium induced hypothyroidism is less common in the presence of antithyroid antibodies.
Ans. False. It is more common.

26. Drug induced anticholinergic effects are grouped under type B adverse reactions.
Ans. False. They are type A adverse reactions.

27. Features of the fetal alcohol syndrome include optic nerve hypoplasia.
Ans. True.

28. Sensitisation to a drug refers to an increase in activity due to repeated application of the drug.
Ans. True.

29. Defective oxidation of drugs involving CYP2D6 is more common in Asians than in Caucasians.
Ans. False. Rates are 1% for Asian and 5% for Caucasians.

30. Psychostimulant drugs display cross sensitization.
Ans. True.

31. Examples of drug induced behavioural teratogenicity include learning disability.
Ans. True.

32. Common psychotropic drug-induced dermatological reactions include exanthematous reactions.
Ans. True.

33. Plasma concentrations of antiparkinsonian drugs are correlated with improvement in psychotic symptoms when treated with neuroleptic drugs.
Ans. False.

34. Antipsychotic drug treatment induces abdominal fat deposition.
Ans. True.

35. A sigmoid dose-response curve of a drug illustrates the dose of the drug required to produce the maximal effect (Emax).
Ans. True.

36. Reported biochemical changes associated with schizophrenia include decreased GABA$_A$ binding sites in cingulate cortex.
Ans. False.

37. The rate of transfer of a drug across the placental barrier is dependent on the concentration gradient between mother and foetus.
Ans. True.

38. Decreased levels of serum aspartate aminotransferase has been associated with treatment with antipsychotic drugs.
Ans. False. Increased levels are associated with this.

39. Hypothermia is a recognised complication of neuroleptic drugs.
Ans. True.

40. Carbamazepine may lower free thyroid hormone concentration.
Ans. True. By increasing the metabolism of the thyroid hormone.

41. It is possible for a patient to have both drug-induced Parkinsonism and Parkinson's disease.
Ans. True.

42. The binding of an antidepressant drug to the 5-HT and NA reuptake sites is most balanced if its NA/5-HT ratio is closest to 1.0.
Ans. True.

43. Antidepressant-induced seizures are more likely to occur in first-born subjects.
Ans. True.

44. Propranolol increases clearance of diazepam.
Ans. False. It decreases this.

45. Antipsychotic drugs block dopamine agonist-induced behaviours in rats, like climbing, eye blink and locomotor activity.
Ans. True.

46. Lithium-induced tremor is more frequent in younger patients than in elderly patients.
Ans. False. It is less frequent in younger patients.

47. Pregabalin binds potently to the alpha-2-delta protein in the brain.
Ans. True.

48. Duloxetine has shown efficacy in the treatment of stress urinary incontinence in women.
Ans. True.

49. Chlorpromazine-related agranulocytosis has been reported to be less common in individuals of Afro-Caribbean ethnic origin.
Ans. False. It is more common in these individuals.

50. Clozapine induces depolarization blockade in the nigrostriatal (A9) neurons.
Ans. False. This occurs in the mesolimbic (A10) neurons.

Paper 39

Questions

1. A drug with a therapeutic window shows sigmoidal dose-response curve. ☐ ☐

2. The risk of upper gastrointestinal haemorrhage is increased in elderly patients who are on SSRIs with a high potency. ☐ ☐

3. Protein kinase C inhibitors have been demonstrated to show antimanic efficacy. ☐ ☐

4. Density of $5HT_2$ receptors is lower in the frontal cortex than in the cerebellum. ☐ ☐

5. Benzodiazepines given during pregnancy can cause low Apgar score. ☐ ☐

6. Clozapine induced agranulocytosis is a type A adverse drug reaction. ☐ ☐

7. Skin pigmentation following prolonged treatment with high doses of phenothiazines is more common in men than in women. ☐ ☐

8. Lorazepam causes retrograde amnesia. ☐ ☐

9. Carbamazepine should not be coadministered with an MAOI. ☐ ☐

10. Withdrawal symptoms on discontinuation of antidepressants are less common in patients with anxiety disorders. ☐ ☐

11. Hepatic enzyme-inducing antiepileptic drugs reduce the efficacy of oral contraceptives in women with epilepsy. ☐ ☐

12. Drug induced allergic reactions are IgE-mediated hypersensitivity reactions. ☐ ☐

13. Recognised side-effects of topiramate include psychosis. ☐ ☐

14. Olanzapine shows selective activation of the c-fos immediate early gene (IEG) in ventral striatum and in medial prefrontal cortex. ☐ ☐

15. Cross-tolerance occurs between LSD and amphetamine type of hallucinogens. ☐ ☐

16. In treatment of schizophrenia, concomitant use of lurasidone with CYP2D6 inhibitors needs no dosage adjustment of lurasidone. ☐ ☐

17. Antidepressants are not recommended for the initial treatment of mild depression. ☐ ☐

18. SSRIs inhibit the uptake of serotonin by platelets. ☐ ☐

19. Type B adverse drug reactions usually have an immunologic mechanism. ☐ ☐

20. Dose-response curve to an agonist in the presence of a competitive antagonist illustrates lowering of the Emax. ☐ ☐

21. Buspirone has no cross-tolerance with benzodiazepines. ☐ ☐

22. Coadministration of lithium and sodium bicarbonate decreases plasma concentration of lithium. ☐ ☐

23. Drug-induced anaphylactoid reactions do not involve IgE production. ☐ ☐

24. Sertraline is contraindicated for initiating antidepressant treatment in patients with ischaemic heart disease. ☐ ☐

25. A small increase in dose of a drug that follows non-linear kinetics can lead to a large increase in plasma concentration. ☐ ☐

26. 4-N-desmethyl olanzapine is an active metabolite of olanzapine. ☐ ☐

27. Pregabalin has no effect on GABAergic mechanisms. ☐ ☐

28. Drugs of lower molecular weight are more likely to produce allergic reactions. ☐ ☐

29. Augmentation of an antidepressant drug with mianserin increases the risk of agranulocytosis. ☐ ☐

30. Antipsychotic drugs devoid of 5-HT$_{2A}$ antagonism include amisulpride. ☐ ☐

31. Alcohol reduces the sedation caused by benzodiazepines. ☐ ☐

32. Chlorpromazine is toxic to bone marrow *in vitro*. ☐ ☐

33. Carbamazepine does not increase plasma level of zopiclone. ☐ ☐

34. Polymorphism of the 5-HT$_{2C}$ receptor gene has been associated with antipsychotic drug-induced weight gain. ☐ ☐

35. A slower rate of absorption is required for hypnotic activity of benzodiazepines. ☐ ☐

36. A teratogenic drug can cause functional abnormalities without causing structural abnormalities in the child. ☐ ☐

37. Drug induced immune complex-mediated membranous glomerulonephritis results in nephrotic syndrome. ☐ ☐

38. The SSRIs have been associated with exacerbation of periodic limb movement disorder. ☐ ☐

39. Survival analysis has shown that on discontinuation of lithium, time to relapse was shorter for depression than for mania. ☐ ☐

40. Chronic use of moclobemide in higher doses produces 20 – 30% inhibition of MAO-B in platelets. ☐ ☐

41. Pregabalin does not bind to plasma proteins. ☐ ☐

42. Coadministration of amiodarone and lithium increases the risk of hypothyroidism. ☐ ☐

43. Dopamine agonists are effective in the treatment of restless legs syndrome and periodic limb movement disorder. ☐ ☐

44. Manifestations of behavioural teratogenicity include learning disability. ☐ ☐

45. Incidence of drug induced adverse cutaneous reactions are more common in women than in men. ☐ ☐

46. The growth hormone response to apomorphine can be used as a measure of serotonin receptor sensitivity. ☐ ☐

47. Most cases of drug-induced granulocytopenia result from bone marrow suppression. ☐ ☐

48. Infants can develop urinary retention and constipation if the mother is taking an anticholinergic drug. ☐ ☐

49. Switching to a second antidepressant produces response in about less than 20% of patients unresponsive to an initial medication trial. ☐ ☐

50. Short acting benzodiazepines have a low volume of distribution. ☐ ☐

Paper 39

1. A drug with a therapeutic window shows sigmoidal dose-response curve.
Ans. **False.** It shows a curvilinear curve.

2. The risk of upper gastrointestinal haemorrhage is increased in elderly patients who are on SSRIs with a high potency.
Ans. **True.**

3. Protein kinase C inhibitors have been demonstrated to show antimanic efficacy.
Ans. **True.**

4. Density of $5HT_2$ receptors is lower in the frontal cortex than in the cerebellum.
Ans. **False.** It is higher in the frontal cortex.

5. Benzodiazepines given during pregnancy can cause low Apgar score.
Ans. **True.**

6. Clozapine induced agranulocytosis is a type A adverse drug reaction.
Ans. **False.** It is a type B reaction.

7. Skin pigmentation following prolonged treatment with high doses of phenothiazines is more common in men than in women.
Ans. **False.** It is more common in women.

8. Lorazepam causes retrograde amnesia.
Ans. **False.** It causes anterograde amnesia.

9. Carbamazepine should not be coadministered with an MAOI.
Ans. **True.**

10. Withdrawal symptoms on discontinuation of antidepressants are less common in patients with anxiety disorders.
Ans. **False.** They are more common in these patients.

11. Hepatic enzyme-inducing antiepileptic drugs reduce the efficacy of oral contraceptives in women with epilepsy.
Ans. **True.**

12. Drug induced allergic reactions are IgE-mediated hypersensitivity reactions.
Ans. **True.**

13. Recognised side-effects of topiramate include psychosis.
Ans. **True.**

14. Olanzapine shows selective activation of the c-fos immediate early gene (IEG) in ventral striatum and in medial prefrontal cortex.
Ans. **True.**

15. Cross-tolerance occurs between LSD and amphetamine type of hallucinogens.
Ans. **False.**

16. In treatment of schizophrenia, concomitant use of lurasidone with CYP2D6 inhibitors needs no dosage adjustment of lurasidone.
Ans. **True.**

17. Antidepressants are not recommended for the initial treatment of mild depression.
Ans. **True.** The risk-benefit ratio is poor.

18. SSRIs inhibit the uptake of serotonin by platelets.
Ans. True.

19. Type B adverse drug reactions usually have an immunologic mechanism.
Ans. True.

20. Dose-response curve to an agonist in the presence of a competitive antagonist illustrates lowering of the Emax.
Ans. False. This is true in the presence of a non-competitive antagonist.

21. Buspirone has no cross-tolerance with benzodiazepines.
Ans. True.

22. Coadministration of lithium and sodium bicarbonate decreases plasma concentration of lithium.
Ans. True.

23. Drug-induced anaphylactoid reactions do not involve IgE production.
Ans. True.

24. Sertraline is contraindicated for initiating antidepressant treatment in patients with ischaemic heart disease.
Ans. False. Sertraline has a strong evidence base for this.

25. A small increase in dose of a drug that follows non-linear kinetics can lead to a large increase in plasma concentration.
Ans. True.

26. 4-N-desmethyl olanzapine is an active metabolite of olanzapine.
Ans. False. It is inactive.

27. Pregabalin has no effect on GABAergic mechanisms.
Ans. True.

28. Drugs of lower molecular weight are more likely to produce allergic reactions.
Ans. False. The opposite is true.

29. Augmentation of an antidepressant drug with mianserin increases the risk of agranulocytosis.
Ans. True.

30. Antipsychotic drugs devoid of 5-HT$_{2A}$ antagonism include amisulpride.
Ans. True.

31. Alcohol reduces the sedation caused by benzodiazepines.
Ans. False. It enhances it by 20 – 30%.

32. Chlorpromazine is toxic to bone marrow *in vitro*.
Ans. True.

33. Carbamazepine does not increase plasma level of zopiclone.
Ans. True. It decreases it by inducing CYP3A4.

34. Polymorphism of the 5-HT$_{2C}$ receptor gene has been associated with antipsychotic drug-induced weight gain.
Ans. True.

35. A slower rate of absorption is required for hypnotic activity of benzodiazepines.
Ans. False. A faster rate is required.

36. A teratogenic drug can cause functional abnormalities without causing structural abnormalities in the child.
Ans. True.

37. Drug induced immune complex-mediated membranous glomerulonephritis results in nephrotic syndrome.

Ans. True.

38. The SSRIs have been associated with exacerbation of periodic limb movement disorder.

Ans. True.

39. Survival analysis has shown that on discontinuation of lithium, time to relapse was shorter for depression than for mania.

Ans. False. It is shorter for mania.

40. Chronic use of moclobemide in higher doses produces 20 – 30% inhibition of MAO-B in platelets.

Ans. True.

41. Pregabalin does not bind to plasma proteins.

Ans. True.

42. Coadministration of amiodarone and lithium increases the risk of hypothyroidism.

Ans. True.

43. Dopamine agonists are effective in the treatment of restless legs syndrome and periodic limb movement disorder.

Ans. True.

44. Manifestations of behavioural teratogenicity include learning disability.

Ans. True.

45. Incidence of drug induced adverse cutaneous reactions are more common in women than in men.

Ans. True.

46. The growth hormone response to apomorphine can be used as a measure of serotonin receptor sensitivity.

Ans. False. It is a measure of dopamine receptor sensitivity.

47. Most cases of drug-induced granulocytopenia result from bone marrow suppression.

Ans. True.

48. Infants can develop urinary retention and constipation if the mother is taking an anticholinergic drug.

Ans. True.

49. Switching to a second antidepressant produces response in about less than 20% of patients unresponsive to an initial medication trial.

Ans. False. It produces a response in 50% of such patients.

50. Short acting benzodiazepines have a low volume of distribution.

Ans. False. They have a high volume of distribution.

Paper 40

	True	False

1. The immune complex mechanism is the most common cause of drug-induced haemolysis. ☐ ☐

2. Patients with HIV have increased sensitivity to neuroleptics resulting in frequent emergence of extra-pyramidal side-effects. ☐ ☐

3. Phase II trials of drug development determine the effects of a new drug with reference to those established drugs in clinical practice. ☐ ☐

4. Sudden discontinuation of antipsychotic drugs can cause tachycardia. ☐ ☐

5. The therapeutic index of a drug is the ratio of its maximum tolerated concentration to its minimum effective concentration. ☐ ☐

6. Pregabalin has shown antipsychotic property in animal models. ☐ ☐

7. Alcohol withdrawal is associated with increased activity in NMDA receptor. ☐ ☐

8. Tolerance to sedative property of antipsychotic drugs generally develops after a few hours. ☐ ☐

9. Fenfluramine has been used as a chemical probe to evaluate the serotonin system. ☐ ☐

10. Cholinesterase inhibitors are antagonised by antimuscarinic drugs. ☐ ☐

11. Fenfluramine causes elevation of prolactin concentration. ☐ ☐

12. Fluoxetine can be used for the treatment of major depressive disorder in children and adolescents under the age of 18. ☐ ☐

13. Increased risk of seizures due to clozapine is independent of its dose. ☐ ☐

14. Ziprasidone is a benzisothiazolyl piperazine. ☐ ☐

15. In treatment with antipsychotic drugs, tolerance usually develops to EPS but not to tardive dyskinesia. ☐ ☐

16. Efficacy of neuroleptic drugs as standard treatment for anorexia nervosa is well established in research. ☐ ☐

17. Antipsychotic drugs with intrinsic anticholinergic properties demonstrate increased risk of causing EPSE. ☐ ☐

18. Factors influencing the teratogenicity include genetic predisposition of the foetus. ☐ ☐

19. Results from flexible dosing drug trials are less clinically representative than the results from fixed-dose trials. ☐ ☐

20. Yohimbine can worsen the core symptoms of post traumatic stress disorder. ☐ ☐

21. The dopamine D3 receptor (DRD3) gene is located on chromosome 16. ☐ ☐

22. Withdrawal of antipsychotic medication in children is more likely to cause tardive dyskinesia than reversible dyskinesia. ☐ ☐

23. Metabolism of ethanol produces a higher plasma concentration of acetaldehyde in Chinese subjects than in Caucasians. ☐ ☐

24. The neuroleptic threshold of haloperidol is close to the dose required for an optimum antipsychotic effect in most patients. ☐ ☐

25. Lithium decreases the release of serotonin from presynaptic terminals. ☐ ☐

26. An effective psychopharmacological intervention in the treatment of generalized anxiety disorder should be continued for at least a year. ☐ ☐

27. Yohimbine infusion does not cause panic in patients with panic disorder. ☐ ☐

28. Benign hyperthermia is a recognised side-effect of clozapine. ☐ ☐

29. Plasma elimination half-lives of renally eliminated drugs are shorter in neonates than in adults. ☐ ☐

30. Oculodermal melanosis has been associated with long-term administration of high doses of phenothiazines. ☐ ☐

31. Methylphenidate blocks the dopamine transporter and increases dopamine levels in the nucleus accumbens. ☐ ☐

32. The dextrorotatory isomer of amphetamine is less potent in behavioural effects than the levorotatory isomer. ☐ ☐

33. Amisulpride has shown efficacy in treatment of primary negative symptoms of schizophrenia. ☐ ☐

34. Benzodiazepine receptor numbers can be measured by PET studies of flumazenil binding. ☐ ☐

35. Alcohol decreases concentrations of plasma endorphins. ☐ ☐

36. Pragmatic clinical trials have more internal validity than randomized controlled trials. ☐ ☐

37. Dantrolene is effective in reducing the muscle rigidity in neuroleptic malignant-syndrome. ☐ ☐

38. Trazodone shows biphasic elimination kinetics. ☐ ☐

39. Oxcarbazepine has reduced risk of causing autoimmune reactions and rashes compared to carbamazepine. ☐ ☐

40. The dopamine receptor agonists are associated with less neuropsychiatric side-effects than levodopa. ☐ ☐

41. A clinical trial is a type of a bioassay involving human subjects. ☐ ☐

42. Phenothiazine induced cholestatic jaundice presents with conjugated hyperbilirubinaemia and increased alkaline phosphase. ☐ ☐

43. Lithium augmentation of ineffective antidepressant treatment has an NNT between 3 and 4. ☐ ☐

44. Mirtazapine reduced the release of noradrenaline by causing the blockade of release-modulating α_2 –adrenoceptors. ☐ ☐

45. Agonists at CCK_B receptors have been demonstrated to be antipanic. ☐ ☐

46. Psychotropic drugs with granulocyte-stimulating effect include lithium. ☐ ☐

47. Alcohol decreases the ability of GABA to open the chloride channel.　☐　☐

48. Increased risk of venous thromboembolism has been associated with treatment with antipsychotic drugs.　☐　☐

49. Fluvoxamine has been demonstrated to be effective in treating obsessive-compulsive disorder in children and adolescents.　☐　☐

50. Controlled studies have shown that children under the age of 18 with anorexia nervosa benefit more from family therapy than from pharmacotherapy.　☐　☐

Paper 40

1. The immune complex mechanism is the most common cause of drug-induced haemolysis.
Ans. True.

2. Patients with HIV have increased sensitivity to neuroleptics resulting in frequent emergence of extra-pyramidal side-effects.
Ans. True.

3. Phase II trials of drug development determine the effects of a new drug with reference to those established drugs in clinical practice.
Ans. False. This happens in phase III trials.

4. Sudden discontinuation of antipsychotic drugs can cause tachycardia.
Ans. False. It can cause bradycardia, due to cholinergic rebound.

5. The therapeutic index of a drug is the ratio of its maximum tolerated concentration to its minimum effective concentration.
Ans. True.

6. Pregabalin has shown antipsychotic property in animal models.
Ans. False. It has shown anxiolytic property.

7. Alcohol withdrawal is associated with increased activity in NMDA receptor.
Ans. True.

8. Tolerance to sedative property of antipsychotic drugs generally develops after a few hours.
Ans. False. It develops in a few weeks.

9. Fenfluramine has been used as a chemical probe to evaluate the serotonin system.
Ans. True.

10. Cholinesterase inhibitors are antagonised by antimuscarinic drugs.
Ans. True.

11. Fenfluramine causes elevation of prolactin concentration.
Ans. True.

12. Fluoxetine can be used for the treatment of major depressive disorder in children and adolescents under the age of 18.
Ans. True.

13. Increased risk of seizures due to clozapine is independent of its dose.
Ans. False.

14. Ziprasidone is a benzisothiazolyl piperazine.
Ans. True.

15. In treatment with antipsychotic drugs, tolerance usually develops to EPS but not to tardive dyskinesia.
Ans. True.

16. Efficacy of neuroleptic drugs as standard treatment for anorexia nervosa is well established in research.
Ans. False.

17. Antipsychotic drugs with intrinsic anticholinergic properties demonstrate increased risk of causing EPSE.
Ans. False. They demonstrate a reduced risk.

18. Factors influencing the teratogenicity include genetic predisposition of the foetus.
Ans. True.

19. Results from flexible dosing drug trials are less clinically representative than the results from fixed-dose trials.
Ans. False. They are more representative.

20. Yohimbine can worsen the core symptoms of post traumatic stress disorder.
Ans. True.

21. The dopamine D3 receptor (DRD3) gene is located on chromosome 16.
Ans. False. Chromosome 3 at 3q13.3.

22. Withdrawal of antipsychotic medication in children is more likely to cause tardive dyskinesia than reversible dyskinesia.
Ans. False. It is less likely.

23. Metabolism of ethanol produces a higher plasma concentration of acetaldehyde in Chinese subjects than in Caucasians.
Ans. True.

24. The neuroleptic threshold of haloperidol is close to the dose required for an optimum antipsychotic effect in most patients.
Ans. True.

25. Lithium decreases the release of serotonin from presynaptic terminals.
Ans. False. It increases this.

26. An effective psychopharmacological intervention in the treatment of generalized anxiety disorder should be continued for at least a year.
Ans. True.

27. Yohimbine infusion does not cause panic in patients with panic disorder.
Ans. False.

28. Benign hyperthermia is a recognised side-effect of clozapine.
Ans. True.

29. Plasma elimination half-lives of renally eliminated drugs are shorter in neonates than in adults.
Ans. False. They are longer in neonates.

30. Oculodermal melanosis has been associated with long-term administration of high doses of phenothiazines.
Ans. True.

31. Methylphenidate blocks the dopamine transporter and increases dopamine levels in the nucleus accumbens.
Ans. True.

32. The dextrorotatory isomer of amphetamine is less potent in behavioural effects than the levorotatory isomer.
Ans. False. More potent.

33. Amisulpride has shown efficacy in treatment of primary negative symptoms of schizophrenia.
Ans. True.

34. Benzodiazepine receptor numbers can be measured by PET studies of flumazenil binding.
Ans. True.

35. Alcohol decreases concentrations of plasma endorphins.
Ans. False. It increases these.

36. Pragmatic clinical trials have more internal validity than randomized controlled trials.
Ans. **False.** They have more external but less internal validity.

37. Dantrolene is effective in reducing the muscle rigidity in neuroleptic malignant-syndrome.
Ans. **True.**

38. Trazodone shows biphasic elimination kinetics.
Ans. **True.**

39. Oxcarbazepine has reduced risk of causing autoimmune reactions and rashes compared to carbamazepine.
Ans. **True.**

40. The dopamine receptor agonists are associated with less neuropsychiatric side-effects than levodopa.
Ans. **False.** More.

41. A clinical trial is a type of a bioassay involving human subjects.
Ans. **True.**

42. Phenothiazine induced cholestatic jaundice presents with conjugated hyperbilirubinaemia and increased alkaline phosphase.
Ans. **True.**

43. Lithium augmentation of ineffective antidepressant treatment has an NNT between 3 and 4.
Ans. **True.**

44. Mirtazapine reduced the release of noradrenaline by causing the blockade of release-modulating α_2 –adrenoceptors.
Ans. **False.** It enhances the release of noradrenaline.

45. Agonists at CCK$_B$ receptors have been demonstrated to be antipanic.
Ans. **False.** They are panicogenic.

46. Psychotropic drugs with granulocyte-stimulating effect include lithium.
Ans. **True.**

47. Alcohol decreases the ability of GABA to open the chloride channel.
Ans. **False.** It increases this.

48. Increased risk of venous thromboembolism has been associated with treatment with antipsychotic drugs.
Ans. **True.**

49. Fluvoxamine has been demonstrated to be effective in treating obsessive-compulsive disorder in children and adolescents.
Ans. **True.**

50. Controlled studies have shown that children under the age of 18 with anorexia nervosa benefit more from family therapy than from pharmacotherapy.
Ans. **True.**

Paper 41

		True	False
1.	Acamprosate increases the power of conditioned aspects of drinking alcohol.	☐	☐
2.	The phenothiazines are contraindicated in the treatment of radiation sickness.	☐	☐
3.	The α-adrenergic receptor blockade by antipsychotic drugs causes pupillary dilatation.	☐	☐
4.	Risk of fatal respiratory depression is high with buprenorphine.	☐	☐
5.	The adverse effects of disulfiram in the absence of alcohol consumption include optic neuritis.	☐	☐
6.	Type II benzodiazepine receptors are associated with muscle relaxant, anxiolytic and anticonvulsant effects.	☐	☐
7.	Neuroleptic malignant syndrome has been described as a type A reaction.	☐	☐
8.	Fixed-dosage drug studies eliminate the effect of differences in prescribing habits among clinicians.	☐	☐
9.	Antidepressant medications have not been shown to be useful when patients with anorexia nervosa are underweight.	☐	☐
10.	Benzodiazepines require GABA to be present for their action.	☐	☐
11.	Stimulant treatment in children has been associated with increased height and weight percentiles with long-term treatment.	☐	☐
12.	Ethanol acts as a blocker of the NMDA channel.	☐	☐
13.	Store-depleting antipsychotics do not cause tardive dyskinesia.	☐	☐
14.	Mirtazapine has been shown to augment SSRIs in unresponsive patients.	☐	☐
15.	Treatment with carbamazepine causes weight gain.	☐	☐
16.	Anandamide activates both cannabinoid and vanilloid receptors.	☐	☐
17.	Phototoxic reactions to drugs have an immunological component.	☐	☐
18.	Reboxetine shows low affinity for the noradrenaline transporter and high affinity for the serotonin transporter.	☐	☐
19.	Depression is a recognised side effect of highly active antiretroviral therapy (HAART).	☐	☐
20.	Inverse agonists at the benzodiazepine site block GABA transmission.	☐	☐
21.	Studies of the discontinuation of lithium treatment for affective disorder suggest that 50% of relapses occur within 10 weeks of stopping treatment.	☐	☐
22.	Riluzole inhibits both the release and the postsynaptic action of glutamate.	☐	☐
23.	Selectivity of an antiparkinsonian drug on muscarinic receptor M1 predicts increased peripheral side effects.	☐	☐
24.	An additive effect between two drugs describes the combined effect of two drugs that is equal to the sum of the effect of each agent given alone.	☐	☐

25. Clozapine is contraindicated in patients receiving protease inhibitors. ☐ ☐

26. Drugs with very short half-life are only useful for sleep induction and not sleep maintenance. ☐ ☐

27. Examples of heterotropic interactions between neurotransmitters include noradrenaline induced inhibition of acetylcholine release. ☐ ☐

28. Bioavailability of a depot antipsychotic drug is lower than with oral preparations. ☐ ☐

29. Tolerance occurs to the effects of benzodiazepines on the waking EEG. ☐ ☐

30. Monitoring of platelet MAO activity is useful in therapeutic monitoring of the reversible inhibitors of MAO-A. ☐ ☐

31. Buprenorphine acts as an antagonist at K opiate receptor. ☐ ☐

32. Brussel sprouts are known to inhibit P450 enzymes. ☐ ☐

33. The ratio of the LD_{50} to the ED_{50} is an indication of how selective a drug is in producing its desired effects relative to its toxicity. ☐ ☐

34. Increased platelet SERT binding has been reported in depressive disorders. ☐ ☐

35. Both typical and atypical neuroleptics have been shown to induce c-fos in nucleus accumbens neurons. ☐ ☐

36. A cost-utility analysis of a drug uses quality adjusted life-years (QALYs) as the expression of the drug's effect. ☐ ☐

37. Benzodiazepines are recommended as primary treatment for longer term treatment of specific phobias. ☐ ☐

38. Picrotoxin acts by blocking the chloride channel associated with the GABA-B receptor. ☐ ☐

39. Recognised effects of reboxetine include attenuation of the pupillary light reflex. ☐ ☐

40. A synergistic effect between two drugs is one in which the combined effect of two drugs is equal to the sum of the effect of each agent given alone. ☐ ☐

41. Antipsychotic drugs have been shown to be more effective treatment for acute forms of schizophrenia than do various types of psychotherapy. ☐ ☐

42. Common side effects of venlafaxine include thrombocytopenia. ☐ ☐

43. Neuropeptide Y is released as a co-transmitter with noradrenaline at many sympathetic nerve endings. ☐ ☐

44. If an antagonist binds at the active site for the agonist, reversible antagonists will be competitive, and irreversible antagonists will be non-competitive. ☐ ☐

45. Neurotensin, an endogenous tridecapeptide, has similar effects to atypical antipsychotic drugs. ☐ ☐

46. Depot preparation of fluphenazine decanoate attains peak plasma levels slower than other depot antipsychotics. ☐ ☐

47. Both benzodiazepines and non-benzodiazepine anxiolytics show marked increase of slow beta waves (12-14 H_z) seen in wake EEG. ☐ ☐

48. Carbamazepine antagonises muscle relaxant effect of non-depolarising muscle relaxants.   ☐   ☐

49. Buspirone is effective in the treatment of acute anxiety.   ☐   ☐

50. Drugs given in solutions of high concentration are absorbed more rapidly than are drugs in solutions of low concentration.   ☐   ☐

Paper 41

1. **Acamprosate increases the power of conditioned aspects of drinking alcohol.**
Ans. **False.**

2. **The phenothiazines are contraindicated in the treatment of radiation sickness.**
Ans. **False.** They are effective in the management of this.

3. **The α-adrenergic receptor blockade by antipsychotic drugs causes pupillary dilatation.**
Ans. **False.** It causes pupillary constriction.

4. **Risk of fatal respiratory depression is high with buprenorphine.**
Ans. **False.** The risk is low.

5. **The adverse effects of disulfiram in the absence of alcohol consumption include optic neuritis.**
Ans. **True.**

6. **Type II benzodiazepine receptors are associated with muscle relaxant, anxiolytic and anticonvulsant effects.**
Ans. **True.**

7. **Neuroleptic malignant syndrome has been described as a type A reaction.**
Ans. **False.** It is a type B reaction.

8. **Fixed-dosage drug studies eliminate the effect of differences in prescribing habits among clinicians.**
Ans. **True.**

9. **Antidepressant medications have not been shown to be useful when patients with anorexia nervosa are underweight.**
Ans. **True.**

10. **Benzodiazepines require GABA to be present for their action.**
Ans. **True.**

11. **Stimulant treatment in children has been associated with increased height and weight percentiles with long-term treatment.**
Ans. **False.** It is associated with decreased height and weight.

12. **Ethanol acts as a blocker of the NMDA channel.**
Ans. **True.**

13. **Store-depleting antipsychotics do not cause tardive dyskinesia.**
Ans. **True.**

14. **Mirtazapine has been shown to augment SSRIs in unresponsive patients.**
Ans. **True.**

15. **Treatment with carbamazepine causes weight gain.**
Ans. **False.**

16. **Anandamide activates both cannabinoid and vanilloid receptors.**
Ans. **True.**

17. **Phototoxic reactions to drugs have an immunological component.**
Ans. **True.**

18. **Reboxetine shows low affinity for the noradrenaline transporter and high affinity for the serotonin transporter.**
Ans. **False.** The opposite is true.

19. Depression is a recognised side effect of highly active antiretroviral therapy (HAART).
Ans. True.

20. Inverse agonists at the benzodiazepine site block GABA transmission.
Ans. False. They decrease GABA transmission.

21. Studies of the discontinuation of lithium treatment for affective disorder suggest that 50% of relapses occur within 10 weeks of stopping treatment.
Ans. True.

22. Riluzole inhibits both the release and the postsynaptic action of glutamate.
Ans. True.

23. Selectivity of an antiparkinsonian drug on muscarinic receptor M1 predicts increased peripheral side effects.
Ans. False. It predicts decreased peripheral side effects.

24. An additive effect between two drugs describes the combined effect of two drugs that is equal to the sum of the effect of each agent given alone.
Ans. True.

25. Clozapine is contraindicated in patients receiving protease inhibitors.
Ans. True.

26. Drugs with very short half-life are only useful for sleep induction and not sleep maintenance.
Ans. True.

27. Examples of heterotropic interactions between neurotransmitters include noradrenaline induced inhibition of acetylcholine release.
Ans. True.

28. Bioavailability of a depot antipsychotic drug is lower than with oral preparations.
Ans. False. It is higher.

29. Tolerance occurs to the effects of benzodiazepines on the waking EEG.
Ans. True.

30. Monitoring of platelet MAO activity is useful in therapeutic monitoring of the reversible inhibitors of MAO-A.
Ans. False. Platelets contain only MAO-B.

31. Buprenorphine acts as an antagonist at K opiate receptor.
Ans. True.

32. Brussel sprouts are known to inhibit P450 enzymes.
Ans. False. They induce them.

33. The ratio of the LD_{50} to the ED_{50} is an indication of how selective a drug is in producing its desired effects relative to its toxicity.
Ans. True.

34. Increased platelet SERT binding has been reported in depressive disorders.
Ans. False. Reduced binding has been reported.

35. Both typical and atypical neuroleptics have been shown to induce c-fos in nucleus accumbens neurons.
Ans. True.

36. A cost-utility analysis of a drug uses quality adjusted life-years (QALYs) as the expression of the drug's effect.
Ans. True.

37. Benzodiazepines are recommended as primary treatment for longer term treatment of specific phobias.

Ans. False.

38. Picrotoxin acts by blocking the chloride channel associated with the GABA-B receptor.

Ans. False. It works on the GABA-A receptor.

39. Recognised effects of reboxetine include attenuation of the pupillary light reflex.

Ans. True.

40. A synergistic effect between two drugs is one in which the combined effect of two drugs is equal to the sum of the effect of each agent given alone.

Ans. False. It is when the combined effect of two drugs is greater than the sum.

41. Antipsychotic drugs have been shown to be more effective treatment for acute forms of schizophrenia than do various types of psychotherapy.

Ans. True.

42. Common side effects of venlafaxine include thrombocytopenia.

Ans. False. It is rare.

43. Neuropeptide Y is released as a co-transmitter with noradrenaline at many sympathetic nerve endings.

Ans. True.

44. If an antagonist binds at the active site for the agonist, reversible antagonists will be competitive, and irreversible antagonists will be non-competitive.

Ans. True.

45. Neurotensin, an endogenous tridecapeptide, has similar effects to atypical antipsychotic drugs.

Ans. True.

46. Depot preparation of fluphenazine decanoate attains peak plasma levels slower than other depot antipsychotics.

Ans. False. Faster (12 – 24 hours).

47. Both benzodiazepines and non-benzodiazepine anxiolytics show marked increase of slow beta waves (12-14 H_z) seen in wake EEG.

Ans. False. Non-benzodiazepine anxiolytics do not show this.

48. Carbamazepine antagonises muscle relaxant effect of non-depolarising muscle relaxants.

Ans. True.

49. Buspirone is effective in the treatment of acute anxiety.

Ans. False.

50. Drugs given in solutions of high concentration are absorbed more rapidly than are drugs in solutions of low concentration.

Ans. True.

Paper 42

		True	False

1. Higher doses of benzodiazepines can depress alveolar ventilation and cause respiratory acidosis. ☐ ☐

2. The atypical neuroleptics induce higher c-fos expression in the dorsolateral striatum. ☐ ☐

3. Family history of bipolar illness is a predictor of good response to lithium. ☐ ☐

4. Tryptophan hydroxylase can be selectively and irreversibly inhibited by ρ-chlorophenylalanine. ☐ ☐

5. Antiparkinsonian drug induced blurring of near vision is caused by paresis of the ciliary muscle. ☐ ☐

6. A first antipsychotic induced acute dystonic reaction is in itself an indication for regular prophylaxis of anticholinergic medication. ☐ ☐

7. Atypical antipsychotics show specific EEG profiles. ☐ ☐

8. Inter individual variations occur in the extent of first-pass metabolism of a given drug. ☐ ☐

9. Biotransformation of a benzodiazepine by oxidation is not impaired in hepatic cirrhosis. ☐ ☐

10. Effects of adenosine receptor agonists include drowsiness and anticonvulsant activity. ☐ ☐

11. Modafinil improves psychomotor performance and vigilance in subjects previously fatigued by sleep deprivation. ☐ ☐

12. After stopping MAOIs, atomoxetine can be started after twelve hours. ☐ ☐

13. Muscarinic antagonists cause amnesia. ☐ ☐

14. Recognised adverse effects of venlafaxine include hyponatraemia. ☐ ☐

15. Diethylthiomethylcarbamate is an active metabolite of disulfiram. ☐ ☐

16. G-protein-coupled 5-HT receptors include 5-HT$_3$ receptor. ☐ ☐

17. Functional antagonism occurs when two drugs produce opposite effects on the same physiological function. ☐ ☐

18. Clozapine does not induce c-fos in the dorsolateral striatum. ☐ ☐

19. 8-hydroxyamoxapine is an active metabolite of amoxapine with potent dopamine antagonist properties. ☐ ☐

20. 5-HT$_{1D}$ receptor agonists are used for treating migraine. ☐ ☐

21. The enzymes involved in phase I reactions of biotransformation of a drug are located mainly in the endoplasmic reticulum. ☐ ☐

22. Neurokinin-1 (NK1) receptor antagonists have demonstrated antidepressant properties. ☐ ☐

23. Risk of psychosis is increased with the concomitant administration of memantine and amantadine. ☐ ☐

	True	False

24. Concomitant use of amisulpride and parenteral erythromycin increases the risk of ventricular arrhythmias. ☐ ☐

25. A drug's ability to cause reduction of the immobility time in forced swim test of an animal is considered as an indication of the drug's potential antipsychotic effect. ☐ ☐

26. Ethanol inhibits NMDA-receptor activation. ☐ ☐

27. The blockade of muscarinic cholinoceptors by a drug can be demonstrated as the antagonism of pilocarpine-evoked miosis. ☐ ☐

28. Methylphenidate was reported to enhance P300 amplitudes in children with attention deficit hyperactivity disorder. ☐ ☐

29. Amisulpride blocks presynaptic D_2 and D_3 autoreceptors at low doses. ☐ ☐

30. SSRIs have been shown to be effective for treating body dysmorphic disorder. ☐ ☐

31. Prolonged apnoea after suxamethonium caused by pseudocholinesterase deficiency is a Mendelian recessive trait. ☐ ☐

32. In treatment resistant patients with schizophrenia, the degree of cerebral ventricular enlargement is unrelated to response to neuroleptics. ☐ ☐

33. Non-competitive antagonists bind at the same site as do the agonists. ☐ ☐

34. Opioid withdrawal syndrome is precipitated by μ-receptor antagonists. ☐ ☐

35. Age-related increase in body fat results in faster elimination of lipid soluble drugs. ☐ ☐

36. The volume of distribution of a drug is decreased in patients with cardiac failure. ☐ ☐

37. Patients with AIDS have been shown to be at reduced risk of developing EPS due to antipsychotic drug treatment. ☐ ☐

38. Anti-obsessional effect of an antidepressant drug takes shorter time to appear than its antidepressant effect. ☐ ☐

39. Antidepressant drugs from different pharmacological classes show a common pattern in pharmaco-EEG studies. ☐ ☐

40. Endogenous tachykinins acting as agonists at NK1 receptor include substance P. ☐ ☐

41. Recognised side effects reported in association with the use of antipsychotics include tardive myoclonus. ☐ ☐

42. Renal tubular function in neonates takes about six weeks to reach adult values. ☐ ☐

43. Drugs that may cause akathisia include calcium channel antagonists. ☐ ☐

44. Plasma half-life of a drug is inversely proportional to the overall rate of clearance of the drug, and directly proportional to the volume of distribution. ☐ ☐

45. The GABA-A receptor is composed of five subunits. ☐ ☐

46. The binding of phenytoin to plasma albumin is increased in nephritic syndrome. ☐ ☐

47. Enkephalinase inhibitors have been shown to cause analgesia without causing dependence. ☐ ☐

48. Inverse agonists at the benzodiazepine receptors are anxiolytic and proconvulsant. ☐ ☐

49. The rapid acetylator phenotype is rare in Inuits and the Japanese. ☐ ☐

50. Benzodiazepines cause a decrease in alpha and beta activity in pharmaco-EEG studies. ☐ ☐

Paper 42

1. Higher doses of benzodiazepines can depress alveolar ventilation and cause respiratory acidosis.

Ans. True.

2. The atypical neuroleptics induce higher c-fos expression in the dorsolateral striatum.

Ans. False. This occurs in the prefrontal cortex.

3. Family history of bipolar illness is a predictor of good response to lithium.

Ans. True.

4. Tryptophan hydroxylase can be selectively and irreversibly inhibited by ρ-chlorophenylalanine.

Ans. True.

5. Antiparkinsonian drug induced blurring of near vision is caused by paresis of the ciliary muscle.

Ans. True.

6. A first antipsychotic induced acute dystonic reaction is in itself an indication for regular prophylaxis of anticholinergic medication.

Ans. False.

7. Atypical antipsychotics show specific EEG profiles.

Ans. False.

8. Inter individual variations occur in the extent of first-pass metabolism of a given drug.

Ans. True.

9. Biotransformation of a benzodiazepine by oxidation is not impaired in hepatic cirrhosis.

Ans. False. Impaired.

10. Effects of adenosine receptor agonists include drowsiness and anticonvulsant activity.

Ans. True.

11. Modafinil improves psychomotor performance and vigilance in subjects previously fatigued by sleep deprivation.

Ans. True.

12. After stopping MAOIs, atomoxetine can be started after twelve hours.

Ans. False. It can be started after two weeks.

13. Muscarinic antagonists cause amnesia.

Ans. True.

14. Recognised adverse effects of venlafaxine include hyponatraemia.

Ans. True.

15. Diethylthiomethylcarbamate is an active metabolite of disulfiram.

Ans. True.

16. G-protein-coupled 5-HT receptors include 5-HT$_3$ receptor.

Ans. False. 5-HT$_3$ is a ligand-gated cation channel.

17. Functional antagonism occurs when two drugs produce opposite effects on the same physiological function.

Ans. True.

18. Clozapine does not induce c-fos in the dorsolateral striatum.

Ans. True.

19. 8-hydroxyamoxapine is an active metabolite of amoxapine with potent dopamine antagonist properties.

Ans. True.

20. 5-HT$_{1D}$ receptor agonists are used for treating migraine.

Ans. True.

21. The enzymes involved in phase I reactions of biotransformation of a drug are located mainly in the endoplasmic reticulum.

Ans. True.

22. Neurokinin-1 (NK1) receptor antagonists have demonstrated antidepressant properties.

Ans. True.

23. Risk of psychosis is increased with the concomitant administration of memantine and amantadine.

Ans. True.

24. Concomitant use of amisulpride and parenteral erythromycin increases the risk of ventricular arrhythmias.

Ans. True.

25. A drug's ability to cause reduction of the immobility time in forced swim test of an animal is considered as an indication of the drug's potential antipsychotic effect.

Ans. False. It is an indication of antidepressant effect.

26. Ethanol inhibits NMDA-receptor activation.

Ans. True.

27. The blockade of muscarinic cholinoceptors by a drug can be demonstrated as the antagonism of pilocarpine-evoked miosis.

Ans. True.

28. Methylphenidate was reported to enhance P300 amplitudes in children with attention deficit hyperactivity disorder.

Ans. True.

29. Amisulpride blocks presynaptic D$_2$ and D$_3$ autoreceptors at low doses.

Ans. True.

30. SSRIs have been shown to be effective for treating body dysmorphic disorder.

Ans. True.

31. Prolonged apnoea after suxamethonium caused by pseudocholinesterase deficiency is a Mendelian recessive trait.

Ans. True.

32. In treatment resistant patients with schizophrenia, the degree of cerebral ventricular enlargement is unrelated to response to neuroleptics.

Ans. True.

33. Non-competitive antagonists bind at the same site as do the agonists.

Ans. False.

34. Opioid withdrawal syndrome is precipitated by μ-receptor antagonists.

Ans. True.

35. Age-related increase in body fat results in faster elimination of lipid soluble drugs.

Ans. True.

36. The volume of distribution of a drug is decreased in patients with cardiac failure.

Ans. True.

37. Patients with AIDS have been shown to be at reduced risk of developing EPS due to antipsychotic drug treatment.
Ans. **False.** They are at increased risk of this.

38. Anti-obsessional effect of an antidepressant drug takes shorter time to appear than its antidepressant effect.
Ans. **False.** It takes longer.

39. Antidepressant drugs from different pharmacological classes show a common pattern in pharmaco-EEG studies.
Ans. **False.**

40. Endogenous tachykinins acting as agonists at NK1 receptor include substance P.
Ans. **True.**

41. Recognised side effects reported in association with the use of antipsychotics include tardive myoclonus.
Ans. **True.**

42. Renal tubular function in neonates takes about six weeks to reach adult values.
Ans. **False.** It takes about 6 months.

43. Drugs that may cause akathisia include calcium channel antagonists.
Ans. **True.**

44. Plasma half-life of a drug is inversely proportional to the overall rate of clearance of the drug, and directly proportional to the volume of distribution.
Ans. **True.**

45. The GABA-A receptor is composed of five subunits.
Ans. **True.** Two $\alpha1$, two $\beta2$ and one $\gamma2$.

46. The binding of phenytoin to plasma albumin is increased in nephritic syndrome.
Ans. **False.** It is reduced.

47. Enkephalinase inhibitors have been shown to cause analgesia without causing dependence.
Ans. **True.**

48. Inverse agonists at the benzodiazepine receptors are anxiolytic and proconvulsant.
Ans. **False.** They are anxiogenic.

49. The rapid acetylator phenotype is rare in Inuits and the Japanese.
Ans. **False.** It is the most common (present in 95%).

50. Benzodiazepines cause a decrease in alpha and beta activity in pharmaco-EEG studies.
Ans. **False.** Increase in beta activity.

Paper 43

Questions

1. Pentazocine can precipitate withdrawal symptoms in morphine-dependent patients. ☐ ☐

2. Substance P antagonist that does not interact with monoamine systems has been shown to be effective as an antidepressant. ☐ ☐

3. Psychosocial treatments are more effective when patients have been stabilised on antipsychotic medication than when they are acutely ill. ☐ ☐

4. Tardive dystonias has been shown to be about twice as common in females as in males. ☐ ☐

5. Area and the curve (AUC) of a drug following its oral administration is similar to as after intravenous administration, if the unmetabolised drug is absorbed completely. ☐ ☐

6. Recognised animal models of depression in behavioural psychopharmacology include tail suspension test. ☐ ☐

7. The colour of the medication has been shown to have no effect on the placebo response. ☐ ☐

8. 5-HT$_3$ receptor antagonists are used as antiemetic drugs. ☐ ☐

9. Withdrawal syndrome following discontinuation of benzodiazepines has been described as type B reaction. ☐ ☐

10. Risk factors for neuroleptic induced akathisia include no previous exposure to neuroleptic drugs. ☐ ☐

11. Paradoxical behavioural responses associated with benzodiazepine treatment include aggression. ☐ ☐

12. Diazepam is more consistently absorbed by intravenous route than intramuscular route. ☐ ☐

13. Tramadol, a metabolite of trazodone, is a weak agonist at μ-opioid receptors. ☐ ☐

14. Rapid acetylator status is an autosomal recessive trait. ☐ ☐

15. Drug related dystonias can present unilaterally. ☐ ☐

16. Cost-effectiveness analysis is used when alternative therapies differ in their clinical effectiveness on a single health outcome, and also differ in costs. ☐ ☐

17. Elimination of methadone can be enhanced by alkaline diuresis. ☐ ☐

18. Acetylation, sulphation and methylation are grouped under Phase 1 reactions of drug metabolism. ☐ ☐

19. Approximately 50% of persons of Mongolian descent have aldehyde dehydrogenase deficiency. ☐ ☐

20. The volume of distribution in infants is increased for water soluble drugs and decreased for lipid soluble drugs. ☐ ☐

21. The severity of the drug withdrawal syndrome is inversely related to the half-life of the drug. ☐ ☐

22. Enzyme inhibition causes increased first-pass metabolism. ☐ ☐

23. Alcohol causes induction of drug metabolism. ☐ ☐

24. Cigarette smoking causes inhibition of CYP2D6. ☐ ☐

25. Symptoms of poisoning by SSRIs include nystagmus. ☐ ☐

26. Intravenous infusion of sodium bicarbonate can arrest arrhythmias caused by tricyclic and related antidepressants. ☐ ☐

27. Activated charcoal is contraindicated in the management of SSRI poisoning. ☐ ☐

28. Flumazenil reverses the opioids effects of dextropropoxyphene. ☐ ☐

29. Pharmacodynamic interactions between two drugs are less predictable than pharmacokinetic interactions. ☐ ☐

30. Sodium oxybate is a central nervous system depressant used for the treatment of narcolepsy with cataplexy. ☐ ☐

31. Atomoxetine is a selective norepinephrine transporter inhibitor. ☐ ☐

32. Plasma membrane transporter facilitates the reuptake of neurotransmitter into presynaptic nerve terminal. ☐ ☐

33. Reboxetine has no effect on major hepatic metabolising enzymes. ☐ ☐

34. Pindolol inhibits the autoinhibition caused by 5-HT1A receptors. ☐ ☐

35. Ketoconazole decreases quetiapine plasma levels. ☐ ☐

36. 5-HT2A antagonists with anti-akasthisia properties include cyproheptadine. ☐ ☐

37. The volume of distribution determines the size of the loading dose of the drug. ☐ ☐

38. Tardive dystonias are responsive to anticholinergic treatment. ☐ ☐

39. Zotepine inhibits norepinephrine reuptake. ☐ ☐

40. Tetrabenazine stimulates vesicular monoamine transporter type 2 (VMAT2). ☐ ☐

41. Recognised causes of depression in a patient with tardive dyskinesia include treatment with tetrabenazine. ☐ ☐

42. Potency of a drug defines the maximum achievable response. ☐ ☐

43. Lithium can worsen antipsychotic induced extra pyramidal syndromes. ☐ ☐

44. Alprazolam is effective for treating bipolar disorder as a monotherapy. ☐ ☐

45. Antidepressants with proven efficacy in premenstrual dysphoric disorder include sertraline. ☐ ☐

46. Both autoreceptors and heteroceptors can either suppress or enhance the release of neurotransmitters. ☐ ☐

47. Neurokinin-1 receptor antagonists have shown antidepressant properties in both forced-swim and tail-suspension tests. ☐ ☐

48. Valproate has affinity for the GABA-A receptor complex. ☐ ☐

49. **The effects of bupropion are mediated by blocking the reuptake of both dopamine and norepinephrine.**   ☐   ☐

50. **At higher doses, moclobemide loses its selectivity for MAO-A.**   ☐   ☐

Paper 43

1. Pentazocine can precipitate withdrawal symptoms in morphine-dependent patients.
Ans. True.

2. Substance P antagonist that does not interact with monoamine systems has been shown to be effective as an antidepressant.
Ans. True.

3. Psychosocial treatments are more effective when patients have been stabilised on antipsychotic medication than when they are acutely ill.
Ans. True.

4. Tardive dystonias has been shown to be about twice as common in females as in males.
Ans. False .

5. Area and the curve (AUC) of a drug following its oral administration is similar to as after intravenous administration, if the unmetabolised drug is absorbed completely.
Ans. True.

6. Recognised animal models of depression in behavioural psychopharmacology include tail suspension test.
Ans. True.

7. The colour of the medication has been shown to have no effect on the placebo response.
Ans. False.

8. $5\text{-}HT_3$ receptor antagonists are used as antiemetic drugs.
Ans. True.

9. Withdrawal syndrome following discontinuation of benzodiazepines has been described as type B reaction.
Ans. False. It is a type E reaction.

10. Risk factors for neuroleptic induced akathisia include no previous exposure to neuroleptic drugs.
Ans. True.

11. Paradoxical behavioural responses associated with benzodiazepine treatment include aggression.
Ans. True.

12. Diazepam is more consistently absorbed by intravenous route than intramuscular route.
Ans. True.

13. Tramadol, a metabolite of trazodone, is a weak agonist at μ-opioid receptors.
Ans. True.

14. Rapid acetylator status is an autosomal recessive trait.
Ans. False. It is autosomal dominant.

15. Drug related dystonias can present unilaterally.
Ans. True.

16. Cost-effectiveness analysis is used when alternative therapies differ in their clinical effectiveness on a single health outcome, and also differ in costs.
Ans. True.

17. Elimination of methadone can be enhanced by alkaline diuresis.
Ans. False. It can be enhanced by acid diuresis.

18. Acetylation, sulphation and methylation are grouped under Phase 1 reactions of drug metabolism.
Ans. False. They are phase II.

19. Approximately 50% of persons of Mongolian descent have aldehyde dehydrogenase deficiency.
Ans. True.

20. The volume of distribution in infants is increased for water soluble drugs and decreased for lipid soluble drugs.
Ans. True.

21. The severity of the drug withdrawal syndrome is inversely related to the half-life of the drug.
Ans. True.

22. Enzyme inhibition causes increased first-pass metabolism.
Ans. False. It causes a decrease.

23. Alcohol causes induction of drug metabolism.
Ans. True. Via induction of CYP2E1.

24. Cigarette smoking causes inhibition of CYP2D6.
Ans. False. It causes inhibition of CYP1A2.

25. Symptoms of poisoning by SSRIs include nystagmus.
Ans. True.

26. Intravenous infusion of sodium bicarbonate can arrest arrhythmias caused by tricyclic and related antidepressants.
Ans. True.

27. Activated charcoal is contraindicated in the management of SSRI poisoning.
Ans. False.

28. Flumazenil reverses the opioids effects of dextropropoxyphene.
Ans. False.

29. Pharmacodynamic interactions between two drugs are less predictable than pharmacokinetic interactions.
Ans. False.

30. Sodium oxybate is a central nervous system depressant used for the treatment of narcolepsy with cataplexy.
Ans. True.

31. Atomoxetine is a selective norepinephrine transporter inhibitor.
Ans. True.

32. Plasma membrane transporter facilitates the reuptake of neurotransmitter into presynaptic nerve terminal.
Ans. True.

33. Reboxetine has no effect on major hepatic metabolising enzymes.
Ans. True.

34. Pindolol inhibits the autoinhibition caused by 5-HT1A receptors.
Ans. True.

35. Ketoconazole decreases quetiapine plasma levels.
Ans. False. It increases it by inhibiting CYP3A4.

36. 5-HT2A antagonists with anti-akasthisia properties include cyproheptadine.
Ans. True.

37. The volume of distribution determines the size of the loading dose of the drug.
Ans. True.

38. Tardive dystonias are responsive to anticholinergic treatment.
Ans. False.

39. Zotepine inhibits norepinephrine reuptake.
Ans. True.

40. Tetrabenazine stimulates vesicular monoamine transporter type 2 (VMAT2).
Ans. False. It inhibits this.

41. Recognised causes of depression in a patient with tardive dyskinesia include treatment with tetrabenazine.
Ans. True.

42. Potency of a drug defines the maximum achievable response.
Ans. False. It is the dose at which responses occur.

43. Lithium can worsen antipsychotic induced extra pyramidal syndromes.
Ans. True.

44. Alprazolam is effective for treating bipolar disorder as a monotherapy.
Ans. False.

45. Antidepressants with proven efficacy in premenstrual dysphoric disorder include sertraline.
Ans. True.

46. Both autoreceptors and heteroceptors can either suppress or enhance the release of neurotransmitters.
Ans. True.

47. Neurokinin-1 receptor antagonists have shown antidepressant properties in both forced-swim and tail-suspension tests.
Ans. True.

48. Valproate has affinity for the GABA-A receptor complex.
Ans. True.

49. The effects of bupropion are mediated by blocking the reuptake of both dopamine and norepinephrine.
Ans. True.

50. At higher doses, moclobemide loses its selectivity for MAO-A.
Ans. True.

Paper 44

		True	False
1.	Strategies to improve medication adherence include cognitive adaptation training.	☐	☐
2.	Vesicular monoamine transporter type 2 (VMAT2) is located on the membrane of the intracellular storage vesicle.	☐	☐
3.	Abrupt discontinuation of an antipsychotic drug can cause dystonia.	☐	☐
4.	Modafinil has no effect on excessive sleepiness in patients with obstructive sleep apnoea/hypopnoea syndrome.	☐	☐
5.	High doses of caffeine can inhibit benzodiazepine receptor binding.	☐	☐
6.	Compliance index is the percentage of the prescribed doses of the medication actually taken by the patient over a specific period.	☐	☐
7.	Phase III drug trials study the toxicological aspects of the drug.	☐	☐
8.	Lithium has cholinomimetic effects.	☐	☐
9.	Alcohol selectively inhibits monoamine oxidase-A in human platelets and brain.	☐	☐
10.	Most neuroleptic sensitivity reactions in Lewy-body dementia occur during the first 2 weeks of treatment.	☐	☐
11.	Acamprosate enhances GABA transmission and antagonises glutamate transmission.	☐	☐
12.	Prostatic hypertrophy worsens antipsychotic-induced urinary retention.	☐	☐
13.	Gabapentin is hydrophilic and readily crosses the blood-brain barrier.	☐	☐
14.	Growth hormone response to clonidine is blunted in major depression.	☐	☐
15.	Antidepressant drug treatment should always be maintained for the duration of the depressive episode.	☐	☐
16.	Increased risk of oral candidiasis is associated with the use of some antipsychotic drugs.	☐	☐
17.	Carbamazepine increases cocaine-mediated dopamine release.	☐	☐
18.	Opiates reduce the perception of peripherally mediated pain.	☐	☐
19.	Pimozide has shown significant efficacy in treatment of delusional disorders.	☐	☐
20.	Noradrenergic tricyclic antidepressant drugs are more effective than serotoninergic tricyclics in treatment of obsessive-compulsive disorder.	☐	☐
21.	Clonazepam is effective in the treatment of REM sleep behaviour disorder.	☐	☐
22.	Decreased cerebrospinal fluid levels of 5-hydroxy-indoleacetic acid are associated with increase in suicidality.	☐	☐
23.	Antipsychotic induced tardive dyskinesia shows more spontaneous remissions in younger patients.	☐	☐
24.	Tardive dyskinesia is a recognised long-term side-effect of lithium.	☐	☐
25.	Raised cortisol output, seen in approximately 50% of patients with major depression, returns to normal in recovery.	☐	☐

26. Pharmacological treatments for PTSD have lower drop-out rates than psychological treatment. ☐ ☐

27. Agitation can cause rapid uptake of a drug given intramuscularly. ☐ ☐

28. A new depressive episode after a 4 – 6 month symptom-free period is considered as a 'relapse'. ☐ ☐

29. Dose-limiting side-effects of MAOI's include ankle oedema. ☐ ☐

30. More lipophilic benzodiazepines are preferable to use in the elderly. ☐ ☐

31. Potent inhibitors of CYP2D6 and CYP3A4 cause increased cholinergic side effects of galantamine. ☐ ☐

32. Moclobemide is contraindicated in patients with phaeochromocytoma. ☐ ☐

33. Elderly individuals are at a greater risk of developing spontaneous dyskinesias independent of antipsychotic drugs. ☐ ☐

34. Sedative antihistamines have the potential for inducing physical dependence. ☐ ☐

35. Carbamazepine induced visual disturbances are dose-related. ☐ ☐

36. Distribution of a drug to the brain is influenced by drug binding to plasma proteins. ☐ ☐

37. Approximately 10% of patients do not respond to therapy with a first-line antidepressant drug. ☐ ☐

38. Tolerance to a drug is not restricted to drugs of abuse. ☐ ☐

39. Low doses of lithium have shown efficacy in the treatment of cyclothymic disorder. ☐ ☐

40. Quetiapine can cause small dose-related decreases in thyroid hormone levels. ☐ ☐

41. Clozapine induced fatal myocarditis is most commonly seen after 6 months of its use. ☐ ☐

42. Most lipophilic drugs become hydrophilic prior to renal excretion. ☐ ☐

43. Drug induced prolongation of the QT interval is associated with increased risk of sudden death. ☐ ☐

44. Delirious patients are less susceptible to parkinsonian side-effects of antipsychotic drugs. ☐ ☐

45. Moclobemide can be used with another antidepressant for augmentation in treatment of resistant depression. ☐ ☐

46. Psychological tolerance to a drug is always associated with its metabolic tolerance. ☐ ☐

47. Doses of SSRIs used for the treatment of obsessive-compulsive disorder (OCD) are lower than those used for treating depression. ☐ ☐

48. Zotepine is contraindicated in acute gout. ☐ ☐

49. Pancreatitis is a common side effect of olanzapine in men. ☐ ☐

50. Amantadine has moderate NMDA receptor blocking properties. ☐ ☐

Paper 44

1. Strategies to improve medication adherence include cognitive adaptation training.
Ans. True.

2. Vesicular monoamine transporter type 2 (VMAT2) is located on the membrane of the intracellular storage vesicle.
Ans. True.

3. Abrupt discontinuation of an antipsychotic drug can cause dystonia.
Ans. True.

4. Modafinil has no effect on excessive sleepiness in patients with obstructive sleep apnoea/hypopnoea syndrome.
Ans. False. It reduces excessive sleepiness.

5. High doses of caffeine can inhibit benzodiazepine receptor binding.
Ans. True.

6. Compliance index is the percentage of the prescribed doses of the medication actually taken by the patient over a specific period.
Ans. True.

7. Phase III drug trials study the toxicological aspects of the drug.
Ans. False. This happens in phase I trials.

8. Lithium has cholinomimetic effects.
Ans. True.

9. Alcohol selectively inhibits monoamine oxidase-A in human platelets and brain.
Ans. False. It inhibits MAO-B.

10. Most neuroleptic sensitivity reactions in Lewy-body dementia occur during the first 2 weeks of treatment.
Ans. True.

11. Acamprosate enhances GABA transmission and antagonises glutamate transmission.
Ans. True.

12. Prostatic hypertrophy worsens antipsychotic-induced urinary retention.
Ans. True.

13. Gabapentin is hydrophilic and readily crosses the blood-brain barrier.
Ans. True.

14. Growth hormone response to clonidine is blunted in major depression.
Ans. True.

15. Antidepressant drug treatment should always be maintained for the duration of the depressive episode.
Ans. True.

16. Increased risk of oral candidiasis is associated with the use of some antipsychotic drugs.
Ans. True. This is due to dry mouth leading to polydypsia.

17. Carbamazepine increases cocaine-mediated dopamine release.
Ans. False. It reduces this.

18. Opiates reduce the perception of peripherally mediated pain.
Ans. False.

19. Pimozide has shown significant efficacy in treatment of delusional disorders.
Ans. True.

20. Noradrenergic tricyclic antidepressant drugs are more effective than serotoninergic tricyclics in treatment of obsessive-compulsive disorder.
Ans. False. The opposite is true.

21. Clonazepam is effective in the treatment of REM sleep behaviour disorder.
Ans. True.

22. Decreased cerebrospinal fluid levels of 5-hydroxy-indoleacetic acid are associated with increase in suicidality.
Ans. True.

23. Antipsychotic induced tardive dyskinesia shows more spontaneous remissions in younger patients.
Ans. True.

24. Tardive dyskinesia is a recognised long-term side-effect of lithium.
Ans. True.

25. Raised cortisol output, seen in approximately 50% of patients with major depression, returns to normal in recovery.
Ans. True.

26. Pharmacological treatments for PTSD have lower drop-out rates than psychological treatment.
Ans. False. The opposite is true.

27. Agitation can cause rapid uptake of a drug given intramuscularly.
Ans. True. This is due to increased blood flow through muscle tissue.

28. A new depressive episode after a 4 – 6 month symptom-free period is considered as a 'relapse'.
Ans. False. It is known as a recurrence.

29. Dose-limiting side-effects of MAOI's include ankle oedema.
Ans. True.

30. More lipophilic benzodiazepines are preferable to use in the elderly.
Ans. False. Less lipophilic benzodiazepines such as lorazepam are preferable.

31. Potent inhibitors of CYP2D6 and CYP3A4 cause increased cholinergic side effects of galantamine.
Ans. True.

32. Moclobemide is contraindicated in patients with phaeochromocytoma.
Ans. True.

33. Elderly individuals are at a greater risk of developing spontaneous dyskinesias independent of antipsychotic drugs.
Ans. True.

34. Sedative antihistamines have the potential for inducing physical dependence.
Ans. False.
35. Carbamazepine induced visual disturbances are dose-related.
Ans. True.

36. Distribution of a drug to the brain is influenced by drug binding to plasma proteins.
Ans. True.

37. Approximately 10% of patients do not respond to therapy with a first-line antidepressant drug.
Ans. False. This is true for around 30% of patients.

38. Tolerance to a drug is not restricted to drugs of abuse.
Ans. True.

39. Low doses of lithium have shown efficacy in the treatment of cyclothymic disorder.

Ans. True.

40. Quetiapine can cause small dose-related decreases in thyroid hormone levels.

Ans. True.

41. Clozapine induced fatal myocarditis is most commonly seen after 6 months of its use.

Ans. False. It is normally seen within the first 2 months.

42. Most lipophilic drugs become hydrophilic prior to renal excretion.

Ans. True. This is via hepatic metabolism.

43. Drug induced prolongation of the QT interval is associated with increased risk of sudden death.

Ans. True.

44. Delirious patients are less susceptible to parkinsonian side-effects of antipsychotic drugs.

Ans. False. They are more susceptible.

45. Moclobemide can be used with another antidepressant for augmentation in treatment of resistant depression.

Ans. False. It should not be taken with other antidepressants.

46. Psychological tolerance to a drug is always associated with its metabolic tolerance.

Ans. False.

47. Doses of SSRIs used for the treatment of obsessive-compulsive disorder (OCD) are lower than those used for treating depression.

Ans. False. Higher doses are used for the treatment of OCD.

48. Zotepine is contraindicated in acute gout.

Ans. True.

49. Pancreatitis is a common side effect of olanzapine in men.

Ans. False. It is very rare.

50. Amantadine has moderate NMDA receptor blocking properties.

Ans. True.

Paper 45

Questions

		True	False
1.	Blunted prolactin response to serotonergic agonists is seen in depressed patients.	☐	☐
2.	Cholinergic antagonists have been associated with improvement in anterograde amnesia.	☐	☐
3.	The antidepressant treatment of dysthymia should continue for more than 2 years.	☐	☐
4.	Increased hip fractures are associated with benzodiazepine use in the elderly.	☐	☐
5.	Ciprofloxacin induces the metabolism of olanzapine.	☐	☐
6.	Lorazepam is metabolised to a pharmacologically inert glucuronide.	☐	☐
7.	5HT1A partial agonism causes down-regulation of auto receptors.	☐	☐
8.	At higher doses, inhibition of noradrenaline and dopamine uptake is seen with SSRI drugs.	☐	☐
9.	Cross-tolerance and cross-dependence can only occur between drugs with a similar mechanism of action at the cellular level.	☐	☐
10.	In the treatment of PTSD symptoms, SSRIs have shown efficacy in improving hyperarousal symptoms but not avoidance.	☐	☐
11.	Some antiparkinsonian drugs can unmask latent tardive dyskinesia.	☐	☐
12.	One out of three patients with depression will respond to placebo.	☐	☐
13.	GABA transporter is located on the postsynaptic side of the GABA synapse.	☐	☐
14.	Sertraline is a weak inhibitor of CYP2D6.	☐	☐
15.	Lithium reduces protein kinase activity.	☐	☐
16.	Acamprosate has disulfiram-like effect in alcohol dependent patients.	☐	☐
17.	Red wine can precipitate hypertensive crisis in a patient with social phobia who is on phenelzine.	☐	☐
18.	Trazodone increases slow wave sleep and has mild REM suppressant effect.	☐	☐
19.	Moclobemide is indicated for the treatment of simple phobia.	☐	☐
20.	If the remission of a depressive episode lasts for 6 weeks, remission is then considered to be recovery.	☐	☐
21.	The direct effects of ligand-gated channels are rapid and transitory.	☐	☐
22.	Valproate increases the expression of the cytoprotective B-cell lymphoma protein Z (Bcl-2).	☐	☐
23.	Recognised side effects of lamotrigine include significant body weight gain.	☐	☐
24.	Tachyphylaxis refers to a rapid decrease in response to a drug.	☐	☐
25.	Lamotrigine dose should be increased if used with valproate.	☐	☐

26. Zotepine can cause dizziness, sedation and hypotension by blocking alpha 1 adrenergic receptors. ☐ ☐

27. The direct effects mediated by G-protein linked receptors are slower in onset and long in duration. ☐ ☐

28. Adding fluoxetine to alprazolam can make the patient very sleepy. ☐ ☐

29. Duloxetine is contraindicated in diabetic peripheral neuropathic pain. ☐ ☐

30. Memantine shows no interactions with cholinesterase inhibitors. ☐ ☐

31. Acetylcholine binds to metabotropic muscarinic receptors and ionotropic nicotinic receptors. ☐ ☐

32. The most common haematological effect of valproate is leukocytosis. ☐ ☐

33. Therapeutic index is directly proportional to the toxic dose of the drug. ☐ ☐

34. Discontinuation of amantadine can trigger neuroleptic malignant syndrome. ☐ ☐

35. Second generation antipsychotics have no risk of tardive dyskinesia. ☐ ☐

36. Antidepressant induced severe hyponatraemia (plasma sodium less than 120 mmol/L) is a medical emergency. ☐ ☐

37. The enzymes that accomplish phase II of drug metabolism include acetyl and glucurony transferases. ☐ ☐

38. Dopamine β hydroxylase gene is located on chromosome 22 q II. ☐ ☐

39. Risk factors for antipsychotic induced dystonia include female gender and older age. ☐ ☐

40. Reboxetine inhibits CYP2D6 and CYP3A4 at high doses. ☐ ☐

41. Valproate has no effect on voltage-sensitive sodium channels. ☐ ☐

42. Sertraline has ability to block dopamine reuptake pump. ☐ ☐

43. Clozapine can be continued in a patient with WBC 2500/mm³ and absolute neutrophil count 1100/mm³. ☐ ☐

44. Lithium blocks the activation of protein kinase by diacylglycerol. ☐ ☐

45. Glutamic acid decarboxylase facilitates the synthesis of glutamic acid from GABA. ☐ ☐

46. In severe congestive heart failure lower drug concentrations will be present in the plasma. ☐ ☐

47. Antipsychotic induced akathisia has both subjective and objective components. ☐ ☐

48. Delay in progression of Alzheimer's disease is evidence of disease-modifying actions of cholinesterase inhibition. ☐ ☐

49. Quetiapine may be the preferred antipsychotic for psychosis in Parkinson's disease. ☐ ☐

50. Sertraline is contraindicated in depressed patients with recent myocardial infarction. ☐ ☐

Paper 45

1. Blunted prolactin response to serotonergic agonists is seen in depressed patients.
Ans. True.

2. Cholinergic antagonists have been associated with improvement in anterograde amnesia.
Ans. False. They cause impairment in anterograde memory.

3. The antidepressant treatment of dysthymia should continue for more than 2 years.
Ans. True.

4. Increased hip fractures are associated with benzodiazepine use in the elderly.
Ans. True.

5. Ciprofloxacin induces the metabolism of olanzapine.
Ans. False. It inhibits it by inhibiting CYP1A2. Improve both.

6. Lorazepam is metabolised to a pharmacologically inert glucuronide.
Ans. True.

7. 5HT1A partial agonism causes down-regulation of auto receptors.
Ans. False. It causes up-regulation of these.

8. At higher doses, inhibition of noradrenaline and dopamine uptake is seen with SSRI drugs.
Ans. True.

9. Cross-tolerance and cross-dependence can only occur between drugs with a similar mechanism of action at the cellular level.
Ans. True.

10. In the treatment of PTSD symptoms, SSRIs have shown efficacy in improving hyperarousal symptoms but not avoidance.
Ans. False. Improve both.

11. Some antiparkinsonian drugs can unmask latent tardive dyskinesia.
Ans. True.

12. One out of three patients with depression will respond to placebo.
Ans. True.

13. GABA transporter is located on the postsynaptic side of the GABA synapse.
Ans. False. It is located on the presynaptic side.

14. Sertraline is a weak inhibitor of CYP2D6.
Ans. True.

15. Lithium reduces protein kinase activity.
Ans. True.

16. Acamprosate has disulfiram-like effect in alcohol dependent patients.
Ans. False.

17. Red wine can precipitate hypertensive crisis in a patient with social phobia who is on phenelzine.
Ans. True.

18. Trazodone increases slow wave sleep and has mild REM suppressant effect.
Ans. True.

19. Moclobemide is indicated for the treatment of simple phobia.
Ans. False. It is indicated for the treatment of social phobia.

20. If the remission of a depressive episode lasts for 6 weeks, remission is then considered to be recovery.
Ans. False. It is considered to be recovery after 6 to 12 months.

21. The direct effects of ligand-gated channels are rapid and transitory.
Ans. True.

22. Valproate increases the expression of the cytoprotective B-cell lymphoma protein Z (Bcl-2).
Ans. True.

23. Recognised side effects of lamotrigine include significant body weight gain.
Ans. False.

24. Tachyphylaxis refers to a rapid decrease in response to a drug.
Ans. True.

25. Lamotrigine dose should be increased if used with valproate.
Ans. False. It should be reduced.

26. Zotepine can cause dizziness, sedation and hypotension by blocking alpha 1 adrenergic receptors.
Ans. True.

27. The direct effects mediated by G-protein linked receptors are slower in onset and long in duration.
Ans. True.

28. Adding fluoxetine to alprazolam can make the patient very sleepy.
Ans. True. Fluoxetine inhibits CYP3A4.

29. Duloxetine is contraindicated in diabetic peripheral neuropathic pain.
Ans. False.

30. Memantine shows no interactions with cholinesterase inhibitors.
Ans. True.

31. Acetylcholine binds to metabotropic muscarinic receptors and ionotropic nicotinic receptors.
Ans. True.

32. The most common haematological effect of valproate is leukocytosis.
Ans. False. The most common effect is thrombocytopenia.

33. Therapeutic index is directly proportional to the toxic dose of the drug.
Ans. True.

34. Discontinuation of amantadine can trigger neuroleptic malignant syndrome.
Ans. True.

35. Second generation antipsychotics have no risk of tardive dyskinesia.
Ans. False.

36. Antidepressant induced severe hyponatraemia (plasma sodium less than 120 mmol/L) is a medical emergency.
Ans. True.

37. The enzymes that accomplish phase II of drug metabolism include acetyl and glucurony transferases.
Ans. True.

38. Dopamine β hydroxylase gene is located on chromosome 22 q II.
Ans. False. It is on chromosome 9 q 34.

39. Risk factors for antipsychotic induced dystonia include female gender and older age.
Ans. False. Male gender and younger age are risk factors.

40. **Reboxetine inhibits CYP2D6 and CYP3A4 at high doses.**
Ans. True.

41. **Valproate has no effect on voltage-sensitive sodium channels.**
Ans. False. It blocks them.

42. **Sertraline has ability to block dopamine reuptake pump.**
Ans. True.

43. **Clozapine can be continued in a patient with WBC 2500/mm³ and absolute neutrophil count 1100/mm³.**
Ans. False. It should be stopped immediately in these circumstances.

44. **Lithium blocks the activation of protein kinase by diacylglycerol.**
Ans. True.

45. **Glutamic acid decarboxylase facilitates the synthesis of glutamic acid from GABA.**
Ans. False. It facilitates the synthesis of glutamic acid to GABA.

46. **In severe congestive heart failure lower drug concentrations will be present in the plasma.**
Ans. False. Drugs are present in a higher concentration in this case.

47. **Antipsychotic induced akathisia has both subjective and objective components.**
Ans. True.

48. **Delay in progression of Alzheimer's disease is evidence of disease-modifying actions of cholinesterase inhibition.**
Ans. False.

49. **Quetiapine may be the preferred antipsychotic for psychosis in Parkinson's disease.**
Ans. True.

50. **Sertraline is contraindicated in depressed patients with recent myocardial infarction.**
Ans. False.

Paper 46

		True	False
1.	Zaleplon is not a benzodiazepine but binds to benzodiazepine receptors.	☐	☐
2.	Cultural factors have no influence on medication adherence.	☐	☐
3.	Valproate inhibits metabolism of lithium.	☐	☐
4.	Flumazenil shows its onset of action in 1 – 2 hours.	☐	☐
5.	Aripiprazole may not only reduce mania but also prevent recurrences of mania in Bipolar Disorder.	☐	☐
6.	Ramelteon binds selectively to melatonin 1 and melatonin 2 receptors as a full agonist.	☐	☐
7.	Modafinil worsens excessive sleepiness in patients with shift-work-sleep disorder.	☐	☐
8.	Weight gain is not common with ziprasidone.	☐	☐
9.	Patients sensitive to the side effects of atomoxetine may include those deficient in CYP2D6.	☐	☐
10.	Scissors gait is a feature of antipsychotic induced dystonia.	☐	☐
11.	More than 40% of quetiapine is excreted unchanged in the urine.	☐	☐
12.	Endozapines that have been isolated from mammalian brain include a diazepam binding inhibitor.	☐	☐
13.	Abrupt withdrawal from alcohol results in decreased REM sleep.	☐	☐
14.	In Asians, the short (s) allele in the serotonin transporter gene is associated with better response to SSRIs.	☐	☐
15.	Pramipexole, a D_2/D_3 receptor agonist, has antidepressant properties.	☐	☐
16.	Reptilian stare is a feature of antipsychotic induced parkinsonism.	☐	☐
17.	Duloxetine has shown efficacy for stress urinary incontinence.	☐	☐
18.	Glycine receptors are voltage-gated ion channels.	☐	☐
19.	The poor metaboliser phenotype for CYP2C19 is common among Asians and rarer in Europenas.	☐	☐
20.	Proinflammatory cytokines can reduce sleep.	☐	☐
21.	Haloperidol shows high affinity for sigmoid receptors in animal models.	☐	☐
22.	Antagonists of the H_1 histamine receptors cause sedation.	☐	☐
23.	The COMT (catechol-O-methyl-transferase) gene is situated on 11p 15.5.	☐	☐
24.	Bonbon sign is a feature of antipsychotic induced tardive dyskinesia.	☐	☐
25.	SSRIs that can cause significant hyper-prolactinaemia include sertraline.	☐	☐
26.	Concomitant use of a CYP3A4 inhibitor drug and pimozide is safe.	☐	☐

27. The number needed to treat (NNT) is the number of patients that need to be treated to prevent one bad outcome compared with a control treatment.   ☐ ☐

28. Ethyleicosapentanoate (E-EPA) can be of benefit in augmenting clozapine in patients refractory to clozapine.   ☐ ☐

29. Risk factors for antipsychotic drug induced tardive dyskinesia include female gender and advancing age.   ☐ ☐

30. Atomoxetine does not have abuse potential.   ☐ ☐

31. Caffeine can reduce seizure length during ECT.   ☐ ☐

32. Drug induced hepatic damage can be due to hypersensitivity reaction to the drug.   ☐ ☐

33. In Caucasians, the long allele in serotonin-promoter gene is associated with an increased probability of response to SSRI's.   ☐ ☐

34. Open clinical trial of a drug usually measures the efficacy of the drug in controls.   ☐ ☐

35. Reversible inhibition of monoamine oxidase type A can be effective in treatment of social anxiety disorder.   ☐ ☐

36. Imipramine has shown efficacy in children with severe form of separation anxiety.   ☐ ☐

37. Pharmacokinetics of ziprasidone is modified by inhibitors and inducers of CYP3A4.   ☐ ☐

38. Branched-chain amino acids can worsen tardive dyskinesia.   ☐ ☐

39. Recent cocaine use increases the risk of antipsychotic-induced dystonias.   ☐ ☐

40. Risk factors for developing QT interval prolongation on the electrocardiogram include methadone.   ☐ ☐

41. The elimination half-life of aripiprazole is shorter than that of clozapine.   ☐ ☐

42. The metabolic ratio (MR) is the urinary ratio between the parent compound and its main metabolite.   ☐ ☐

43. SSRIs may reduce the risk of upper gastrointestinal bleeding.   ☐ ☐

44. Power of the study is reduced if there is a large response in the placebo group of an antidepressant drug trial.   ☐ ☐

45. Chewing betel nuts has been associated with opposing the actions of the anticholinergic procyclidine.   ☐ ☐

46. Lithium induced hypothyroidism is rarer in men than in women.   ☐ ☐

47. The addictive potential of a drug increases with its receptor affinity.   ☐ ☐

48. Levodopa is converted in the body, firstly to norepinephrine and then to dopamine.   ☐ ☐

49. Steady state levels of olanzapine are reached within 2 days of starting treatment.   ☐ ☐

50. Complications of methadone overdose include rhabdomyolysis.   ☐ ☐

Paper 46

1. Zaleplon is not a benzodiazepine but binds to benzodiazepine receptors.
Ans. True.

2. Cultural factors have no influence on medication adherence.
Ans. False.

3. Valproate inhibits metabolism of lithium.
Ans. False. It has no pharmacokinetic interactions with lithium.

4. Flumazenil shows its onset of action in 1 – 2 hours.
Ans. False. It takes 1 – 2 minutes.

5. Aripiprazole may not only reduce mania but also prevent recurrences of mania in Bipolar Disorder.
Ans. True.

6. Ramelteon binds selectively to melatonin 1 and melatonin 2 receptors as a full agonist.
Ans. True.

7. Modafinil worsens excessive sleepiness in patients with shift-work-sleep disorder.
Ans. False. It reduces this.

8. Weight gain is not common with ziprasidone.
Ans. True.

9. Patients sensitive to the side effects of atomoxetine may include those deficient in CYP2D6.
Ans. True.

10. Scissors gait is a feature of antipsychotic induced dystonia.
Ans. True.

11. More than 40% of quetiapine is excreted unchanged in the urine.
Ans. False. Less than 5% is unchanged.

12. Endozapines that have been isolated from mammalian brain include a diazepam binding inhibitor.
Ans. True.

13. Abrupt withdrawal from alcohol results in decreased REM sleep.
Ans. False. REM rebound occurs.

14. In Asians, the short (s) allele in the serotonin transporter gene is associated with better response to SSRIs.
Ans. True.

15. Pramipexole, a D_2/D_3 receptor agonist, has antidepressant properties.
Ans. True.

16. Reptilian stare is a feature of antipsychotic induced parkinsonism.
Ans. True.

17. Duloxetine has shown efficacy for stress urinary incontinence.
Ans. True.

18. Glycine receptors are voltage-gated ion channels.
Ans. False. They are ligand-gated.

19. The poor metaboliser phenotype for CYP2C19 is common among Asians and rarer in Europenas.
Ans. True. It occurs in around 20% of Asians 3 – 5% of Europeans.

20. Proinflammatory cytokines can reduce sleep.

Ans. False. They can induce sleep.

21. Haloperidol shows high affinity for sigmoid receptors in animal models.

Ans. True.

22. Antagonists of the H_1 histamine receptors cause sedation.

Ans. True.

23. The COMT (catechol-O-methyl-transferase) gene is situated on 11p 15.5.

Ans. False. It is on 22q11.11 – q11.2.

24. Bonbon sign is a feature of antipsychotic induced tardive dyskinesia.

Ans. True.

25. SSRIs that can cause significant hyper-prolactinaemia include sertraline.

Ans. False.

26. Concomitant use of a CYP3A4 inhibitor drug and pimozide is safe.

Ans. False. It is contraindicated.

27. The number needed to treat (NNT) is the number of patients that need to be treated to prevent one bad outcome compared with a control treatment.

Ans. True.

28. Ethyleicosapentanoate (E-EPA) can be of benefit in augmenting clozapine in patients refractory to clozapine.

Ans. True.

29. Risk factors for antipsychotic drug induced tardive dyskinesia include female gender and advancing age.

Ans. True.

30. Atomoxetine does not have abuse potential.

Ans. True.

31. Caffeine can reduce seizure length during ECT.

Ans. False. It can reduce this.

32. Drug induced hepatic damage can be due to hypersensitivity reaction to the drug.

Ans. True.

33. In Caucasians, the long allele in serotonin-promoter gene is associated with an increased probability of response to SSRI's.

Ans. True.

34. Open clinical trial of a drug usually measures the efficacy of the drug in controls.

Ans. False. No controls are used in this type of trial.

35. Reversible inhibition of monoamine oxidase type A can be effective in treatment of social anxiety disorder.

Ans. True.

36. Imipramine has shown efficacy in children with severe form of separation anxiety.

Ans. True.

37. Pharmacokinetics of ziprasidone is modified by inhibitors and inducers of CYP3A4.

Ans. True.

38. Branched-chain amino acids can worsen tardive dyskinesia.

Ans. False. They can reduce it.

39. Recent cocaine use increases the risk of antipsychotic-induced dystonias.

Ans. True.

40. Risk factors for developing QT interval prolongation on the electrocardiogram include methadone.

Ans. True.

41. The elimination half-life of aripiprazole is shorter than that of clozapine.

Ans. False. Aripiprazole half-life=75 hrs , clozapine half-life=12hrs.

42. The metabolic ratio (MR) is the urinary ratio between the parent compound and its main metabolite.

Ans. True.

43. SSRIs may reduce the risk of upper gastrointestinal bleeding.

Ans. False.

44. Power of the study is reduced if there is a large response in the placebo group of an antidepressant drug trial.

Ans. True.

45. Chewing betel nuts has been associated with opposing the actions of the anticholinergic procyclidine.

Ans. True. This is because betel nuts contain arecoline.

46. Lithium induced hypothyroidism is rarer in men than in women.

Ans. True.

47. The addictive potential of a drug increases with its receptor affinity.

Ans. False.

48. Levodopa is converted in the body, firstly to norepinephrine and then to dopamine.

Ans. False. It is converted to dopamine first.

49. Steady state levels of olanzapine are reached within 2 days of starting treatment.

Ans. False. After 7 days.

50. Complications of methadone overdose include rhabdomyolysis.

Ans. True.

Paper 47

		True	False
1.	Presence of borderline personality disorder predicts a poorer outcome in treatment of depression with antidepressants.	☐	☐
2.	Placebo response rates are high in older people.	☐	☐
3.	Non-opioid analgesics are preferred to opioid analgesics for analgesia for buprenorphine-prescribed patients.	☐	☐
4.	Latin square design is applied in situations where more than two treatment conditions are being evaluated.	☐	☐
5.	Valproic acid can cause reversible hair loss in 10% of patients.	☐	☐
6.	Olanzapine pharmacokinetics are different in different ethnic groups.	☐	☐
7.	Carbamazepine should be avoided in individuals presenting with HIV with mania.	☐	☐
8.	Lithium is usually discontinued 24 hours pre-operatively before major surgery.	☐	☐
9.	In treatment of depression in children and adolescents, fluoxetine should be considered as first-line treatment.	☐	☐
10.	Contraindications to use disulfiram include coronary artery disease.	☐	☐
11.	SSRIs have been shown to attenuate the panic attacks occurring in CO_2 and cholecystokinin challenge paradigms.	☐	☐
12.	Epileptic seizures are a recognised complication of intravenous use of pure heroin.	☐	☐
13.	The pharmacokinetics of quetiapine are mainly affected by inducers or inhibitors of CYP1A2.	☐	☐
14.	Clonidine has been found to be effective in the treatment of attention deficit hyperactivity disorder.	☐	☐
15.	Risk of non-discrimination between drug and placebo is reduced if patients with mild depression are included in the study.	☐	☐
16.	Withdrawal delirium is a recognised feature of amphetamine abuse.	☐	☐
17.	Dose-titration studies are a closer reflection of actual clinical practice compared to fixed-dose studies.	☐	☐
18.	Acamprosate and disulfiram have no interactions when given together.	☐	☐
19.	Caucasian patient populations require lower doses of antipsychotic drugs compared with oriental population.	☐	☐
20.	Bupropion is a selective norepinephrine dopamine reuptake inhibitor.	☐	☐
21.	Kinaesthetic hallucinations may be experienced in benzodiazepine withdrawal.	☐	☐
22.	Recommended treatments for neuroleptic malignant syndrome include dopamine antagonists.	☐	☐
23.	The scopolamine challenge paradigm is used for the investigation of impairment of attention and memory.	☐	☐

24. Memantine is not effective in improving cognition in cerebrovascular disorder. ☐ ☐

25. The administration of nicotine reduces dopamine levels in the prefrontal cortex. ☐ ☐

26. The anxiolytic effect of diazepam is reduced by caffeine. ☐ ☐

27. All atypical antipsychotics display fast dissociation from the D_2 receptor. ☐ ☐

28. Homovanillic acid is a metabolite of serotonin. ☐ ☐

29. Norcocaine is less cardiotoxic than cocaine. ☐ ☐

30. Opioid withdrawal in the first trimester is associated with miscarriage. ☐ ☐

31. Antipsychotics are the drugs of choice for catatonia. ☐ ☐

32. Acetylcholinesterase inhibitors are associated with rare incidence of sinus bradycardia. ☐ ☐

33. Lithium augmentation of ineffective antidepressant treatment has an NNT between 7 and 8. ☐ ☐

34. The glutamatergic hypothesis suggests that a hypoglutamatergic state at postsynaptic NMDA receptors causes psychosis. ☐ ☐

35. Drop-out rates of patients due to inadequate efficacy of the drug are low in fixed-dose studies. ☐ ☐

36. Antipsychotic induced akathisia is associated with suicidality. ☐ ☐

37. Zolpidem is contraindicated during breast-feeding. ☐ ☐

38. Magnetic resonance spectroscopy can be used to study the effects of psychotropic drugs on brain neurochemistry. ☐ ☐

39. Tricyclic antidepressant drugs increase the reuptake of dopamine to the presynaptic neuron by the dopamine transporter protein. ☐ ☐

40. Neurokinin -1 receptor antagonists have shown efficacy in the treatment of depressive disorders. ☐ ☐

41. Indole-containing vegetables like cabbage and cauliflower down regulate CYP1A activity. ☐ ☐

42. Tricyclic antidepressants can be effective in the treatment of neuropathic pain. ☐ ☐

43. Placebo response is generally evident much later than the usual response to a drug. ☐ ☐

44. List of drugs frequently causing hypo-oestrogenaemia includes aripiprazole. ☐ ☐

45. Memantine does not affect the inhibition of acetylcholinesterase by donepezil. ☐ ☐

46. Mescaline and psyloscibin are inverse agonists at 5HT2A receptors. ☐ ☐

47. Cannabinoid receptors are not present in the immune system. ☐ ☐

48. Alcohol enhances inhibitory neurotransmission at GABA-A receptors and reduces the excitatory neurotransmission at the N-methyl-d-aspartate (NMDA) receptor. ☐ ☐

49. **Cytochrome P450 isoenzymes are located in mitochondria.** ☐ ☐

50. **Buspiroine, ipsapirone and gepirone are 5HT 1A receptor partial agonists and act as anxiolytics.** ☐ ☐

Paper 47

1. **Presence of borderline personality disorder predicts a poorer outcome in treatment of depression with antidepressants.**
Ans. True.

2. **Placebo response rates are high in older people.**
Ans. False. They are higher in younger people.

3. **Non-opioid analgesics are preferred to opioid analgesics for analgesia for buprenorphine-prescribed patients.**
Ans. True.

4. **Latin square design is applied in situations where more than two treatment conditions are being evaluated.**
Ans. True.

5. **Valproic acid can cause reversible hair loss in 10% of patients.**
Ans. True.

6. **Olanzapine pharmacokinetics are different in different ethnic groups.**
Ans. False.

7. **Carbamazepine should be avoided in individuals presenting with HIV with mania.**
Ans. True. This is due to its interactions with retrovirals.

8. **Lithium is usually discontinued 24 hours pre-operatively before major surgery.**
Ans. True.

9. **In treatment of depression in children and adolescents, fluoxetine should be considered as first-line treatment.**
Ans. False. Psychological treatments should be considered first.

10. **Contraindications to use disulfiram include coronary artery disease.**
Ans. True.

11. **SSRIs have been shown to attenuate the panic attacks occurring in CO_2 and cholecystokinin challenge paradigms.**
Ans. True.

12. **Epileptic seizures are a recognised complication of intravenous use of pure heroin.**
Ans. False.

13. **The pharmacokinetics of quetiapine are mainly affected by inducers or inhibitors of CYP1A2.**
Ans. False. They are affected by inducers and inhibitors of CYP3A4.

14. **Clonidine has been found to be effective in the treatment of attention deficit hyperactivity disorder.**
Ans. True.

15. **Risk of non-discrimination between drug and placebo is reduced if patients with mild depression are included in the study.**
Ans. False.

16. **Withdrawal delirium is a recognised feature of amphetamine abuse.**
Ans. False.

17. **Dose-titration studies are a closer reflection of actual clinical practice compared to fixed-dose studies.**
Ans. True.

18. Acamprosate and disulfiram have no interactions when given together.
Ans. True.

19. Caucasian patient populations require lower doses of antipsychotic drugs compared with oriental population.
Ans. False. They require higher doses.

20. Bupropion is a selective norepinephrine dopamine reuptake inhibitor.
Ans. True.

21. Kinaesthetic hallucinations may be experienced in benzodiazepine withdrawal.
Ans. True.

22. Recommended treatments for neuroleptic malignant syndrome include dopamine antagonists.
Ans. False.

23. The scopolamine challenge paradigm is used for the investigation of impairment of attention and memory.
Ans. True.

24. Memantine is not effective in improving cognition in cerebrovascular disorder.
Ans. False.

25. The administration of nicotine reduces dopamine levels in the prefrontal cortex.
Ans. False.

26. The anxiolytic effect of diazepam is reduced by caffeine.
Ans. True.

27. All atypical antipsychotics display fast dissociation from the D_2 receptor.
Ans. False.

28. Homovanillic acid is a metabolite of serotonin.
Ans. False. It is a metabolite of dopamine.

29. Norcocaine is less cardiotoxic than cocaine.
Ans. False. It is more cardiotoxic.

30. Opioid withdrawal in the first trimester is associated with miscarriage.
Ans. True.

31. Antipsychotics are the drugs of choice for catatonia.
Ans. False. Benzodiazepines are used.

32. Acetylcholinesterase inhibitors are associated with rare incidence of sinus bradycardia.
Ans. True.

33. Lithium augmentation of ineffective antidepressant treatment has an NNT between 7 and 8.
Ans. False. It is between 3 and 4.

34. The glutamatergic hypothesis suggests that a hypoglutamatergic state at postsynaptic NMDA receptors causes psychosis.
Ans. True.

35. Drop-out rates of patients due to inadequate efficacy of the drug are low in fixed-dose studies.
Ans. False.

36. Antipsychotic induced akathisia is associated with suicidality.
Ans. True.

37. Zolpidem is contraindicated during breast-feeding.
Ans. False.

38. **Magnetic resonance spectroscopy can be used to study the effects of psychotropic drugs on brain neurochemistry.**
Ans. **True.**

39. **Tricyclic antidepressant drugs increase the reuptake of dopamine to the presynaptic neuron by the dopamine transporter protein.**
Ans. **False.** They inhibit dopamine reuptake.

40. **Neurokinin -1 receptor antagonists have shown efficacy in the treatment of depressive disorders.**
Ans. **True.**

41. **Indole-containing vegetables like cabbage and cauliflower down regulate CYP1A activity.**
Ans. **False.** They up regulate this.

42. **Tricyclic antidepressants can be effective in the treatment of neuropathic pain.**
Ans. **True.**

43. **Placebo response is generally evident much later than the usual response to a drug.**
Ans. **False.** It is generally earlier.

44. **List of drugs frequently causing hypo-oestrogenaemia includes aripiprazole.**
Ans. **False.**

45. **Memantine does not affect the inhibition of acetylcholinesterase by donepezil.**
Ans. **True.**

46. **Mescaline and psyloscibin are inverse agonists at 5HT2A receptors.**
Ans. **False.** They are partial agonists.

47. **Cannabinoid receptors are not present in the immune system.**
Ans. **False.**

48. **Alcohol enhances inhibitory neurotransmission at GABA-A receptors and reduces the excitatory neurotransmission at the N-methyl-d-aspartate (NMDA) receptor.**
Ans. **True.**

49. **Cytochrome P450 isoenzymes are located in mitochondria.**
Ans. **False.** They are in the endoplasmic reticulum.

50. **Buspiroine, ipsapirone and gepirone are 5HT 1A receptor partial agonists and act as anxiolytics.**
Ans. **True.**

Paper 48

Questions

	True	False

1. Stress- induced hypothermia test is used in animal models of anxiety to study the anxiolytic effects of a drug.

2. Poor metabolizers of a drug do not show the signs of toxicity during treatment with standard doses.

3. Cocaine inhibits the dopamine reuptake transporter protein.

4. Reversible neutropaenia occurs in 15% of clozapine- treated patients.

5. Actions of asenapine include alpha-1 adrenergic antagonism.

6. The rate- corrected QT can be calculated by dividing the actual QT by the square root of the RR interval (both measured in seconds).

7. A multiple fixed- dose study design of a drug has the risk of false negative judgement.

8. Carriers of multiduplicated functional CYP2D6 alleles are known to demonstrate ultra rapid drug metabolism.

9. Intramuscular diazepam is highly recommended for rapid tranquilization in the management of acute schizophrenia.

10. Metabotropic melatonin MT1, and MT2 receptors are present in the suprachiasmatic nucleus.

11. Naltrexone produces a toxic reaction like antabuse if alcohol is used concurrently.

12. Diazepam can cause anterograde amnesia.

13. Natural neurotransmitters are full agonists.

14. Patients recruited into clinical trials by advertisement may show higher placebo response rates than the spontaneously booked patients in the out patient clinics.

15. Abnormal involuntary movement scale is a self- report questionnaire.

16. Examples of G- protein coupled receptors include glutamate receptors.

17. SSRIs are not effective for the treatment of body dysmorphic disorder.

18. Lithium toxicity can be precipitated by angiotensin- converting enzyme inhibitors.

19. The norepinephrine transporter (NET) has the affinity for the transport of both norepinerphrine and dopamine.

20. 5HT2A antagonist actions of an antipsychotic causes hyperprolactinemia.

21. Placebo treatments are not used to study the effects of discontinuation or withdrawl symptoms of a drug.

22. The effect of iloperidone on the QT interval may be augmented by paroxetine.

23. Trazadone is safer than sertraline for the treatment of depression following recent myocardial infarction.

24. When directly compared antipsychotic drug treatment is associated with greater benefit than ECT in treatment of schizophrenia.

25. The dopamine D4 receptor (DRD4) gene is located on the short arm of chromosome 11 at 11p15.5.

26. Ketamine acts as an agonist at the NMDA receptors.

27. Loratidine is a histamine (H1) antagonist.

28. The treatment of bipolar depression with lamotrigine increases the risk of switching to manic phase.

29. The elimination of olanzapine is complete after four weeks after the last injection of olanzapine pamoate.

30. Low dose antipsychotics can reduce stereotypies in patients with learning disabilities.

31. Rimonabant is a selective cannabinoid CB1 receptor antagonist which has shown efficacy in smoking cessation.

32. Naloxone acts as a partial opioid agonist.

33. The dopamine transporter (DAT) has high affinity for the transport of both dopamine and amphetamines.

34. Natural endogenous neurotransmitters are full agonists.

35. In crossover designs pharmacological carryover effects between two drugs can be reduced by inserting a placebo period after the first treatment.

36. Pregabalin targets voltage sensitive sodium channels.

37. 5HTIA and 5HT2A receptors have similar actions in regulating dopamine release.

38. Rivastigmine is a pseudo- irreversible non- competitive inhibitor of acetylcholinesterase.

39. Oprenolol is a partial agonist at the D2 receptor.

40. Bupropion is a noradrenaline and serotonin reuptake inhibitor.

41. Quetiapine has shown efficacy as monotherapy in bipolar I and bipolar II depression.

42. Phase I drug metabolising enzymes include cytochrome P450.

43. Chronic antidepressant treatment decreases the activity of cAMP response element binding protein (CREB) in cerebral limbic structures.

44. Dosage of iloperidone should be reduced by one-half when administered with clarithromycin.

45. Sodium valproate induced adverse effects include hypoammonaemia.

46. Symptoms of venlafaxine overdose may include seizures.

47. Opioid withdrawl in the third trimester is associated with premature labour and fetal death.

48. **The serotonin transporter (SERT) has high affinity for the transport of ecstacy.** ☐ ☐

49. **Ramelteon is an MT1 and MT2 receptor antagonist.** ☐ ☐

50. **Renal failure secondary to rhabdomyolysis is the usual cause of death in neuroleptic malignant syndrome.** ☐ ☐

1. Stress- induced hypothermia test is used in animal models of anxiety to study the anxiolytic effects of a drug.
Ans. True.

2. Poor metabolizers of a drug do not show the signs of toxicity during treatment with standard doses.
Ans. False. They may show the signs.

3. Cocaine inhibits the dopamine reuptake transporter protein.
Ans. True.

4. Reversible neutropaenia occurs in 15% of clozapine- treated patients.
Ans. False. It occurs in around 3% of these patients.

5. Actions of asenapine include alpha-1 adrenergic antagonism.
Ans. True.

6. The rate- corrected QT can be calculated by dividing the actual QT by the square root of the RR interval (both measured in seconds).
Ans. True. It is known as Bazett's formula.

7. A multiple fixed- dose study design of a drug has the risk of false negative judgement.
Ans. True.

8. Carriers of multiduplicated functional CYP2D6 alleles are known to demonstrate ultra rapid drug metabolism.
Ans. True.

9. Intramuscular diazepam is highly recommended for rapid tranquilization in the management of acute schizophrenia.
Ans. False.

10. Metabotropic melatonin MT1, and MT2 receptors are present in the suprachiasmatic nucleus.
Ans. True.

11. Naltrexone produces a toxic reaction like antabuse if alcohol is used concurrently.
Ans. False.

12. Diazepam can cause anterograde amnesia.
Ans. True.

13. Natural neurotransmitters are full agonists.
Ans. True.

14. Patients recruited into clinical trials by advertisement may show higher placebo response rates than the spontaneously booked patients in the out patient clinics.
Ans. True.

15. Abnormal involuntary movement scale is a self- report questionnaire.
Ans. False. It is a clinician rated scale.

16. Examples of G- protein coupled receptors include glutamate receptors.
Ans. True.

17. SSRIs are not effective for the treatment of body dysmorphic disorder.
Ans. False.

18. Lithium toxicity can be precipitated by angiotensin- converting enzyme inhibitors.
Ans. True.

19. The norepinephrine transporter (NET) has the affinity for the transport of both norepinerphrine and dopamine.
Ans. True.

20. 5HT2A antagonist actions of an antipsychotic causes hyperprolactinemia.
Ans. False. It reduces hyperprolactinemia.

21. Placebo treatments are not used to study the effects of discontinuation or withdrawl symptoms of a drug.
Ans. False.

22. The effect of iloperidone on the QT interval may be augmented by paroxetine.
Ans. True. Paroxetine is a cyp2d6 inhibitor.

23. Trazadone is safer than sertraline for the treatment of depression following recent myocardiac infarction.
Ans. False. Sertraline is safer.

24. When directly compared antipsychotic drug treatment is associated with greater benefit than ECT in treatment of schizophrenia.
Ans. True.

25. The dopamine D4 receptor (DRD4) gene is located on the short arm of chromosome 11 at 11p15.5.
Ans. True.

26. Ketamine acts as an agonist at the NMDA receptors.
Ans. False. It acts as an antagonist.

27. Loratidine is a histamine (H1) antagonist.
Ans. True.

28. The treatment of bipolar depression with lamotrigine increases the risk of switching to manic phase.
Ans. False.

29. The elimination of olanzapine is complete after four weeks after the last injection of olanzapine pamoate.
Ans. False. It takes approximately six to eight months.

30. Low dose antipsychotics can reduce stereotypies in patients with learning disabilities.
Ans. True.

31. Rimonabant is a selective cannabinoid CB1 receptor antagonist which has shown efficacy in smoking cessation.
Ans. True.

32. Naloxone acts as a partial opioid agonist.
Ans. False. It acts as a competitive antagonist.

33. The dopamine transporter (DAT) has high affinity for the transport of both dopamine and amphetamines.
Ans. True.

34. Natural endogenous neurotransmitters are full agonists.
Ans. True.

35. In crossover designs pharmacological carryover effects between two drugs can be reduced by inserting a placebo period after the first treatment.
Ans. True.

36. Pregabalin targets voltage sensitive sodium channels.
Ans. False. It targets voltage sensitive calcium channels.

37. 5HTIA and 5HT2A receptors have similar actions in regulating dopamine release.
Ans. False. Opposite actions (5HT2A inhibits DA).

38. Rivastigmine is a pseudo- irreversible non- competitive inhibitor of acetylcholinesterase.
Ans. True.

39. Oprenolol is a partial agonist at the D2 receptor.
Ans. False. It is at the beta-adrenoceptor.

40. Bupropion is a noradrenaline and serotonin reuptake inhibitor.
Ans. False. It is a noradrenaline and dopamine reuptake inhibitor.

41. Quetiapine has shown efficacy as monotherapy in bipolar I and bipolar II depression.
Ans. True.

42. Phase I drug metabolising enzymes include cytochrome P450.
Ans. True.

43. Chronic antidepressant treatment decreases the activity of cAMP response element binding protein (CREB) in cerebral limbic structures.
Ans. False. It increases this.

44. Dosage of iloperidone should be reduced by one-half when administered with clarithromycin.
Ans. True. Because clarithromycin is a cyp3a4 inhibitor.

45. Sodium valproate induced adverse effects include hypoammonaemia.
Ans. False. They include hyperammonaemia.

46. Symptoms of venlafaxine overdose may include seizures.
Ans. True.

47. Opioid withdrawl in the third trimester is associated with premature labour and fetal death.
Ans. True.

48. The serotonin transporter (SERT) has high affinity for the transport of ecstacy.
Ans. True.

49. Ramelteon is an MT1 and MT2 receptor antagonist.
Ans. False. It is an agonist.

50. Renal failure secondary to rhabdomyolysis is the usual cause of death in neuroleptic malignant syndrome.
Ans. True.

Paper 49

	True	False

1. Fatal toxicity index is a measure of the number of overdose deaths per million prescriptions. ☐ ☐

2. Elevation of plasma levels of one drug by another drug is a pharmacodynamic interaction. ☐ ☐

3. Lithium induced neutrophilia is not dose related. ☐ ☐

4. Venlafaxine shows differential affinity for the 5HT and noradrenaline transporter proteins at different doses. ☐ ☐

5. Memantine does not affect the inhibition of acetylcholinesterase by donepezil. ☐ ☐

6. Muscarinic receptors M1 and M2 inhibit cAMP. ☐ ☐

7. Fluoxetine has been associated with improved insulin sensitivity in obese patients with non- insulin dependant diabetes. ☐ ☐

8. Oxybutynin may be effective in children with treatment- resistant nocturnal enuresis caused by detrusor instability. ☐ ☐

9. Lamotrigine targets voltage sensitive calcium channels. ☐ ☐

10. Dopamine release is disinhibited by 5HT2A antagonism in nigrostriatal pathway. ☐ ☐

11. The peak plasma level (cMax) of a drug is reached when the rates of absorption and elimination are equal. ☐ ☐

12. More than 30% of all serotonin in the body is found in the CNS. ☐ ☐

13. Lithium decreases cholinergic activity in the brain. ☐ ☐

14. Pharmacokinetics of asenapine are similar in patients with severe renal impairment and patients with no renal impairment. ☐ ☐

15. Serotonin increases prolactin release by stimulating 5HT2A receptors. ☐ ☐

16. Hydroxybupropion is an inactive metabolite of bupropion. ☐ ☐

17. Cocaine binds with high affinity to transporter molecules for 5HT, DA and norepinephrine. ☐ ☐

18. Elimination half- life of dopamine is approximately 2 hours. ☐ ☐

19. Varenicline is a selective alpha 4 beta 2 nicotinic acetylcholine receptor partial agonist. ☐ ☐

20. Methylphenidate blocks both dopamine transporter (DAT) and norepinephrine transporter (NET). ☐ ☐

21. Antidepressant dose for prophylaxis in adults is one third of the dose used for acute treatment. ☐ ☐

22. Signs of opioid neonatal syndrome include autonomic hyperactivity. ☐ ☐

23. Methadone may cause hallucinations. ☐ ☐

24. Dopamine readily crosses blood- brain- barrier. ☐ ☐

	True	False

25. Glycine is synthesised in the brain from L- serine by serine hydroxymethyl- transferase. ☐ ☐

26. Seizures are recognized features of LSD withdrawal. ☐ ☐

27. Atomoxetine is a norepinephrine transporter inhibitor (NET). ☐ ☐

28. Isothiocyanate containing vegetables like watercress can inhibit CYP2E1. ☐ ☐

29. Congenital physical anomalies due to inutero cocaine exposure often include ocular and urogenital systems. ☐ ☐

30. Alzheimer's disease is associated with increased activity of choline acetyltranserase. ☐ ☐

31. Buproprion is contraindicated in patients with history of seizures. ☐ ☐

32. 5HT3 receptor is a G- Protein coupled receptor. ☐ ☐

33. Lamotrigine is commonly associated with cell-mediated type 4 allergic reactions. ☐ ☐

34. Treatment with SSRIs in patients with PTSD is associated with improvement in concurrent depression but not in core PTSD symptoms. ☐ ☐

35. Both SSRI and SNRI groups of antidepressant drugs are absorbed from the proximal small intestine. ☐ ☐

36. Transdermal drug absorption is increased in the elderly population. ☐ ☐

37. Blockade of both H1 and 5HT2C receptors is associated with increased weight gain. ☐ ☐

38. Concomitant use of amantadine and memantine increases the risk of psychosis. ☐ ☐

39. Observational trials are performed during phase III clinical development. ☐ ☐

40. Lithium is effective in reducing the self injurious behaviour in patients with learning disability. ☐ ☐

41. Chlorpromazine inhibits CYP2D6 and CYPIA2. ☐ ☐

42. Venlafaxine blocks reuptake of noradrenaline at doses below 150mg. ☐ ☐

43. Stimulant drugs have smaller effect sizes for reducing ADHD symptoms than selective norepinephrine reuptake inhibitors. ☐ ☐

44. Response to treatment with acetylcholinesterase inhibitors is seen only in cognitive impairment but not in functional impairment. ☐ ☐

45. Bupropion should not be prescribed patients with a history of seizures. ☐ ☐

46. Garlic is an inducer of CYP3A4 and inhibitor of CYP2E1. ☐ ☐

47. List of antipsychotic drugs with no significant effect on QTc interval include aripiprazole. ☐ ☐

48. Acidification of urine increases the excretion rate of phencyclidine. ☐ ☐

49. Enantiomers of a drug always show similar drug profiles. ☐ ☐

50. Phase IV clinical trials are undertaken in less stringently defined groups of the patients than used in phase III clinical trials. ☐ ☐

1. **Fatal toxicity index is a measure of the number of overdose deaths per million prescriptions.**
Ans. True.

2. **Elevation of plasma levels of one drug by another drug is a pharmacodynamic interaction.**
Ans. False. It is a pharmacokinetic interaction.

3. **Lithium induced neutrophilia is not dose related.**
Ans. True.

4. **Venlafaxine shows differential affinity for the 5HT and noradrenaline transporter proteins at different doses.**
Ans. True.

5. **Memantine does not affect the inhibition of acetlycholinesterase by donepezil.**
Ans. True.

6. **Muscarinic receptors M1 and M2 inhibit cAMP.**
Ans. False. M1, M3 and M5 activate IP3, M2 and M4 inhibit cAMP.

7. **Fluoxetine has been associated with improved insulin sensitivity in obese patients with non- insulin dependant diabetes.**
Ans. True.

8. **Oxybutynin may be effective in children with treatment- resistant nocturnal enuresis caused by detrusor instability.**
Ans. True.

9. **Lamotrigine targets voltage sensitive calcium channels.**
Ans. False. It targets voltage sensitive sodium channels.

10. **Dopamine release is disinhibited by 5HT2A antagonism in nigrostriatal pathway.**
Ans. True.

11. **The peak plasma level (cMax) of a drug is reached when the rates of absorption and elimination are equal.**
Ans. True.

12. **More than 30% of all serotonin in the body is found in the CNS.**
Ans. False. Less than 2 %.

13. **Lithium decreases cholinergic activity in the brain.**
Ans. False.

14. **Pharmacokinetics of asenapine are similar in patients with severe renal impairment and patients with no renal impairment.**
Ans. True.

15. **Serotonin increases prolactin release by stimulating 5HT2A receptors.**
Ans. True.

16. **Hydroxybupropion is an inactive metabolite of bupropion.**
Ans. False. It is an active metabolite.

17. **Cocaine binds with high affinity to transporter molecules for 5HT, DA and norepinephrine.**
Ans. True.

18. **Elimination half- life of dopamine is approximately 2 hours.**
Ans. False. It is eliminated in approximately 2 minutes.

19. Varenicline is a selective alpha 4 beta 2 nicotinic acetylcholine receptor partial agonist.
Ans. True. It is effective in smoking cessation.

20. Methylphenidate blocks both dopamine transporter (DAT) and norepinephrine transporter (NET).
Ans. True.

21. Antidepressant dose for prophylaxis in adults is one third of the dose used for acute treatment.
Ans. False. It is the same dose.

22. Signs of opioid neonatal syndrome include autonomic hyperactivity.
Ans. True.

23. Methadone may cause hallucinations.
Ans. True.

24. Dopamine readily crosses blood- brain- barrier.
Ans. False.

25. Glycine is synthesised in the brain from L- serine by serine hydroxymethyl- transferase.
Ans. True.

26. Seizures are recognized features of LSD withdrawal.
Ans. False. LSD does not cause physical dependence.

27. Atomoxetine is a norepinephrine transporter inhibitor (NET).
Ans. True.

28. Isothiocyanate containing vegetables like watercress can inhibit CYP2E1.
Ans. True.

29. Congenital physical anomalies due to inutero cocaine exposure often include ocular and urogenital systems.
Ans. True.

30. Alzheimer's disease is associated with increased activity of choline acetyltranserase.
Ans. False. It is associated with reduced activity.

31. Buproprion is contraindicated in patients with history of seizures.
Ans. True.

32. 5HT3 receptor is a G- Protein coupled receptor.
Ans. False. It is a ligand gated ion channel.

33. Lamotrigine is commonly associated with cell-mediated type 4 allergic reactions.
Ans. True.

34. Treatment with SSRIs in patients with PTSD is associated with improvement in concurrent depression but not in core PTSD symptoms.
Ans. False. It improves both.

35. Both SSRI and SNRI groups of antidepressant drugs are absorbed from the proximal small intestine.
Ans. True.

36. Transdermal drug absorption is increased in the elderly population.
Ans. False. It is diminished in the elderly.

37. Blockade of both H1 and 5HT2C receptors is associated with increased weight gain.
Ans. True.

38. Concomitant use of amantadine and memantine increases the risk of psychosis.
Ans. True.

39. Observational trials are performed during phase III clinical development.
Ans. **False.** They are preformed during phase IV.

40. Lithium is effective in reducing the self injurious behaviour in patients with learning disability.
Ans. **True.**

41. Chlorpromazine inhibits CYP2D6 and CYPIA2.
Ans. **True.**

42. Venlafaxine blocks reuptake of noradrenaline at doses below 150mg.
Ans. **False.** It blocks the reuptake of serotonin.

43. Stimulant drugs have smaller effect sizes for reducing ADHD symptoms than selective norepinephrine reuptake inhibitors.
Ans. **False.** The opposite is true.

44. Response to treatment with acetylcholinesterase inhibitors is seen only in cognitive impairment but not in functional impairment.
Ans. **False.** It is seen in both.

45. Bupropion should not be prescribed patients with a history of seizures.
Ans. **True.**

46. Garlic is an inducer of CYP3A4 and inhibitor of CYP2E1.
Ans. **True.**

47. List of antipsychotic drugs with no significant effect on QTc interval include aripiprazole.
Ans. **True.**

48. Acidification of urine increases the excretion rate of phencyclidine.
Ans. **True.**

49. Enantiomers of a drug always show similar drug profiles.
Ans. **True.**

50. Phase IV clinical trials are undertaken in less stringently defined groups of the patients than used in phase III clinical trials.
Ans. **True.**

Paper 50

		True	False
1.	Plasma protein binding for venlafaxine is greater than for duloxetine.	☐	☐
2.	Naltrexone reduces the number of drinking drugs during the maintenance phase of alcohol abstinence.	☐	☐
3.	Exposure to SSRIs in late pregnancy is associated with increased risk of persistent pulmonary hypertension of the newborn.	☐	☐
4.	Plasma concentration of reboxetine is correlated with its antidepressant action.	☐	☐
5.	Carbamazepine reduces clearance of olanzapine.	☐	☐
6.	2 milligrams of haloperidol can induce more than 70% striatal D2 occupancy.	☐	☐
7.	Lithium inhibits the action of antidiuretic hormone on the kidney.	☐	☐
8.	Ser9Gly polymorphism of the DRD3 gene has been associated with dystonia.	☐	☐
9.	Naloxone and naltrexone have no intrinsic activity at the mu opioid receptor.	☐	☐
10.	The intravenous preparation of citalopram has been shown to be effective in the treatment of depression.	☐	☐
11.	Phase 2 drug metabolising enzymes include N-acetyltransferase.	☐	☐
12.	Escitalopram binds to an allostreric site on the transporter protein.	☐	☐
13.	Discontinuation of pregabalin leads to clinically significant withdrawal syndrome.	☐	☐
14.	Response to one mood stabiliser is predictive of a response to another mood stabiliser.	☐	☐
15.	Clozapine induced ECG changes include ST depression.	☐	☐
16.	Allosteric modulators have no activity of their own.	☐	☐
17.	Venlafaxine is associated with greater toxicity in overdose than SSRIs.	☐	☐
18.	SSRIs reduce attentional vigilance to threat- related stimuli.	☐	☐
19.	Coadministration of aripiprazole with valproate will decrease the concentration of aripiprazole.	☐	☐
20.	Partial agonists can be agonists or antagonists at receptors.	☐	☐
21.	Both lithium and valproate increase the brain derived neurotrophic factor (BDNF).	☐	☐
22.	Sertraline is associated with higher risk of diarrhoea than other SSRIs.	☐	☐
23.	Aripiprazole is associated with increased risk of dyslipidaemia.	☐	☐
24.	AMPA receptors mediate fast excitatory synaptic transmission.	☐	☐
25.	A polymorphism within the serotonin transporter gene (SERTPR) has been associated with response to SSRIs treatment.	☐	☐
26.	Zaleplon increases sleep onset latency.	☐	☐
27.	Milnacipran blocks norepinephrine and 5HT reuptake with equal affinity.	☐	☐

28. Lithium protects against clozapine induced agranulocytosis. ☐ ☐

29. Cross- titration of antipsychotic drugs is more likely to cause relapse than other methods of switching. ☐ ☐

30. Kynurenic acid is a non- selective antagonist of excitatory amino acid receptors. ☐ ☐

31. Buprenorphine produces higher risk of respiratory depression than methadone. ☐ ☐

32. Adding memantine to a cholinesterase inhibitor has shown efficacy in the treatment of dementia. ☐ ☐

33. The ratio of dextrorphan/dextromethorphan (DX/DM) is a marker of CYP2D6 activity. ☐ ☐

34. Acamprosate is a metabotropic glutamate receptor 5 (mGluR5) agonist. ☐ ☐

35. Valproate induces the uridine diphosphate glucuronosyl transferase. ☐ ☐

36. Debrisoquine can be used as a probe to determine the CYP2D6 status of an individual. ☐ ☐

37. Venous thromboembolism has been associated with clozapine. ☐ ☐

38. Neonatal signs after late in-utero exposure to SSRIs include hypertonia. ☐ ☐

39. Eszopiclone is effective for the long term treatment of insomnia. ☐ ☐

40. Quetiapine blocks the decreases in hippocampal BDNF that occur with stress. ☐ ☐

41. Older individuals have lower intracellular lithium levels than younger individuals. ☐ ☐

42. Oral hypoaesthesia is a recognised side effect of asenapine. ☐ ☐

43. Magnesium is a positive allosteric modulator at NMDA glutamate receptors. ☐ ☐

44. Naringinin , a constituent of processed grapefruit juice , is known to inhibit CYP3A4. ☐ ☐

45. Asians exhibit more CYP2C19 polymorphisms than CYP2D6 polymorphisms. ☐ ☐

46. Hypotonia is a recognised feature of serotonergic syndrome. ☐ ☐

47. The rate of titration of lamotrigine should be halved when coadministered with valproate. ☐ ☐

48. Rifampicin causes a significant decrease in the clearance of diazepam. ☐ ☐

49. Competitive inhibitors of CYP1A2 include caffeine. ☐ ☐

50. Persistence is the duration of time from initiation to discontinuation of treatment. ☐ ☐

Paper 50

1. **Plasma protein binding for venlafaxine is greater than for duloxetine.**
Ans. **False.** Greater for duloxetine.

2. **Naltrexone reduces the number of drinking drugs during the maintenance phase of alcohol abstinence.**
Ans. **True.**

3. **Exposure to SSRIs in late pregnancy is associated with increased risk of persistent pulmonary hypertension of the newborn.**
Ans. **True.**

4. **Plasma concentration of reboxetine is correlated with its antidepressant action.**
Ans. **False.**

5. **Carbamazepine reduces clearance of olanzapine.**
Ans. **False.** It increases it.

6. **2 milligrams of haloperidol can induce more than 70% striatal D2 occupancy.**
Ans. **True.**

7. **Lithium inhibits the action of antidiuretic hormone on the kidney.**
Ans. **True.**

8. **Ser9Gly polymorphism of the DRD3 gene has been associated with dystonia.**
Ans. **False.** Associated with tardive dyskinesia.

9. **Naloxone and naltrexone have no intrinsic activity at the mu opioid receptor.**
Ans. **True.**

10. **The intravenous preparation of citalopram has been shown to be effective in the treatment of depression.**
Ans. **True.**

11. **Phase 2 drug metabolising enzymes include N-acetyltransferase.**
Ans. **True.**

12. **Escitalopram binds to an allostreric site on the transporter protein.**
Ans. **True.**

13. **Discontinuation of pregabalin leads to clinically significant withdrawal syndrome.**
Ans. **False.**

14. **Response to one mood stabiliser is predictive of a response to another mood stabiliser.**
Ans. **False.**

15. **Clozapine induced ECG changes include ST depression.**
Ans. **True.**

16. **Allosteric modulators have no activity of their own.**
Ans. **True.**

17. **Venlafaxine is associated with greater toxicity in overdose than SSRIs.**
Ans. **True.**

18. **SSRIs reduce attentional vigilance to threat- related stimuli.**
Ans. **True.**

19. **Coadministration of aripiprazole with valproate will decrease the concentration of aripiprazole.**
Ans. **False.** No significant effect.

20. Partial agonists can be agonists or antagonists at receptors.
Ans. True.

21. Both lithium and valproate increase the brain derived neurotrophic factor (BDNF).
Ans. True.

22. Sertraline is associated with higher risk of diarrhoea than other SSRIs.
Ans. True.

23. Aripiprazole is associated with increased risk of dyslipidaemia.
Ans. False.

24. AMPA receptors mediate fast excitatory synaptic transmission.
Ans. True.

25. A polymorphism within the serotonin transporter gene (SERTPR) has been associated with response to SSRIs treatment.
Ans. True.

26. Zaleplon increases sleep onset latency.
Ans. False. It decreases this.

27. Milnacipran blocks norepinephrine and 5HT reuptake with equal affinity.
Ans. True.

28. Lithium protects against clozapine induced agranulocytosis.
Ans. False.

29. Cross- titration of antipsychotic drugs is more likely to cause relapse than other methods of switching.
Ans. False. It is less likely to cause relapse.

30. Kynurenic acid is a non- selective antagonist of excitatory amino acid receptors.
Ans. True. It is neuroprotective.

31. Buprenorphine produces higher risk of respiratory depression than methadone.
Ans. False. It carries a lower risk.

32. Adding memantine to a cholinesterase inhibitor has shown efficacy in the treatment of dementia.
Ans. True.

33. The ratio of dextrorphan/dextromethorphan (DX/DM) is a marker of CYP2D6 activity.
Ans. True.

34. Acamprosate is a metabotropic glutamate receptor 5 (mGluR5) agonist.
Ans. False. It is an antagonist.

35. Valproate induces the uridine diphosphate glucuronosyl transferase.
Ans. False. It inhibits this.

36. Debrisoquine can be used as a probe to determine the CYP2D6 status of an individual.
Ans. True

37. Venous thromboembolism has been associated with clozapine.
Ans. True.

38. Neonatal signs after late in-utero exposure to SSRIs include hypertonia.
Ans. True.

39. Eszopiclone is effective for the long term treatment of insomnia.
Ans. True.

40. **Quetiapine blocks the decreases in hippocampal BDNF that occur with stress.**
Ans. **True.**

41. **Older individuals have lower intracellular lithium levels than younger individuals.**
Ans. **False.** They have higher levels.

42. **Oral hypoaesthesia is a recognised side effect of asenapine.**
Ans. **True.**

43. **Magnesium is a positive allosteric modulator at NMDA glutamate receptors.**
Ans. **False.** It is a negative allosteric modulator.

44. **Naringinin , a constituent of processed grapefruit juice , is known to inhibit CYP3A4.**
Ans. **True.**

45. **Asians exhibit more CYP2C19 polymorphisms than CYP2D6 polymorphisms.**
Ans. **True.**

46. **Hypotonia is a recognised feature of serotonergic syndrome.**
Ans. **False.** Rigidity and hyperreflexiaare recognised features.

47. **The rate of titration of lamotrigine should be halved when coadministered with valproate.**
Ans. **True.**

48. **Rifampicin causes a significant decrease in the clearance of diazepam.**
Ans. **False.** It causes an increase.

49. **Competitive inhibitors of CYP1A2 include caffeine.**
Ans. **True.**

50. **Persistence is the duration of time from initiation to discontinuation of treatment.**
Ans. **True.**

Paper 51

1. **Common side-effects of SSRIs include the following except:**

a) Nausea
b) Paraesthesia
c) Abdominal pain
d) Diarrhoea
e) Sexual dysfunction

2. **Identify the false statement regarding antidepressant drugs:**

a) Any individual drug may not be effective.
b) The antidepressant effect does not occur immediately.
c) Craving, tolerance and addiction do not occur.
d) Persistent adverse effects do not occur.
e) Patients with recurrent depression should not stop antidepressants before 2 years.

3. **Peripheral antimuscarinic effects of the antipsychotic drugs include the following except:**
a) Dry mouth
b) Blurred vision
c) Urinary retention
d) Constipation
e) Pyrexia

4. **The antidopaminergic action of the AP drugs on the tuberoinfundibular pathway results in the following except:**

a) Galactorrhoea
b) Gynaecomastia
c) Akathisia
d) Menstrual abnormalities
e) Reduced libido

5. **Pharmacodynamic drug interactions include the following except:**

a) Enzyme induction
b) Interaction at receptors
c) Synergisms
d) Inhibition of drug transport
e) Inhibition of drug uptake

6. **Signs of lithium intoxication include the following except:**

a) Dysarthria
b) Coarse tremor
c) Drowsiness
d) Lens opacity
e) Vomiting

7. Identify the false statement about plasma level determinations of the psychotropic drugs:

a) Useful if toxicity is suspected.
b) Useful if drug interactions are suspected.
c) Useful if the drug has a narrow therapeutic index.
d) Useful if target levels are established.
e) Useful if assessed after 5 doses.

8. Identify the false statement regarding risperidone long acting injection:

a) It is not an esterified form of the drug.
b) A test dose is not required.
c) Therapeutic levels reach after one week after the first injection.
d) It must be administered every two weeks.
e) Less than 10% experience EPSE.

9. Risk of seizures is high with the following except:

a) Moclobemide
b) Clomipramine
c) Clozapine
d) Zotepine
e) Dosulepine

10. Depression is a recognised side effect of the following except:

a) Vigabatrin
b) Gabapentin
c) Tiagabine
d) Topiramate
e) Valproate

11. Risks of using SSRIs in pregnancy include the following except:

a) Increased rate of spontaneous abortions.
b) Increased risk of persistent pulmonary hypertension of the newborn.
c) Low scores of early APGAR.
d) Increased agitation and irritability in neonates.
e) Increased neural tube defects

12. Lithium use in pregnancy is associated with the following in the neonate except:

a) Goitre
b) Hypertonia
c) Ebstein's anomaly
d) Arrhythmias
e) Rash

13. Dosage reduction is recommended in hepatic impairment for the following except

a) Amisulpride
b) Quetiapine
c) Aripiprazole
d) Clozapine
e) Risperidone

14. Which of the following is preferably avoided if glomerular filtration rate is <10ml/min:

   a) Haloperidol
   b) Valproate
   c) Lamotrigine
   d) Lithium
   e) Olanzapine

15. Zuclopenthixol acetate should not be used for the following except:

   a) Patients who are neuroleptic naive.
   b) Patients who are sensitive to EPSE.
   c) Patients who accept oral medication.
   d) Patients with cardiac disease.
   e) Patients who require repeated injections of short acting antipsychotic drugs.

16. Identify the false statement regarding caffeine:

   a) Metabolised by CYP1A2.
   b) Can inhibit benzodiazepine receptor binding.
   c) Increases clozapine plasma levels.
   d) Decreases clearance of lithium.
   e) An established withdrawal syndrome exists.

17. Drugs that can cause 'antabuse' reaction with alcohol include the following except:

   a) Grieseofulvin
   b) Metronidazole
   c) Isosorbide dinitrate
   d) Disulfiram
   e) Aspirin

18. Side-effects of reboxetine include the following except:

   a) Urinary hesitancy
   b) Blurred vision
   c) Headache
   d) Dry mouth
   e) Nasal decongestion

19. Animal models used in testing the efficacy of antidepressants include the following except:

   a) Forced swim test
   b) Tail suspension test
   c) Learned helplessnss test
   d) Chronic mild stress model
   e) Pre pulse inhibition

20. Predictors of good response to lithium include the following except:

   a) Mania followed by depression
   b) Family history of bipolar illness
   c) Previous good response to treatment
   d) Rapid cycling bipolar illness
   e) Greter adherence to treatment

21. Action of sodium valproate include the following except:

a) Enhances GABA-transaminase
b) Increase GABA binding in hippocampus
c) Inhibits the formation of protein kinase C
d) Reduces the action of NA at alpha2 receptors
e) Enhances GABAergic function

22. Lithium has shown efficacy in the following conditions except:

a) Reversal of neutropenia
b) Reduction in impulsivity
c) Adjunct to antipsychotics in schizophrenia
d) Prophylaxis in schizoaffective disorder
e) Adjunct to antidepressants in general anxiety disorder

23. Identify the false statement regarding benzodiazepines:

a) In the absence of GABA , BZD will have no effect of their own.
b) Inverse agonists at the BZD receptor enhance the action of GABA.
c) BDZs reduce REM sleep.
d) Tolerance to EEG effects occurs.
e) Withdrawal syndrome can not be treated by 5HT1a partial agonists.

24. Placebo response is common in the following except:

a) Anxiety disorders
b) Manic episodes
c) Dissociative states
d) Dementia
e) Drug-induced psychosis

25. All but one of the following increase the risk of antidepressant induced hyponatraemia:

a) Old age
b) Female sex
c) Obesity
d) GFR<50ml/min
e) SSRIs

26. Following antidepressant drugs are relatively safe in diabetes except:

a) Fluoxetine
b) Duloxetine
c) MAOI
d) Sertraline
e) Reboxetine

27. Identify the antidepressant which is contraindicated in recent MI:

a) Sertraline
b) Moclobemide
c) Fluoxetine
d) Amitriptyline
e) Mirtazapine

28. Side effects due to muscarinic cholinergic blockade include the following except:

a) Urinary retention
b) Blurred vision
c) Weight gain
d) Tachycardia
e) Dry mouth

29. Identify the approximate 5HT2A: D2 affinity ratio of clozapine from the following:

a) 10: 1
b) 8: 1
c) 30: 1
d) 5: 1
e) 1: 1

30. Indications for treatment with antidepressant drugs include the following except:

a) Post-traumatic stress disorder
b) Social phobia
c) Bulimia nervosa
d) Dissociative disorder
e) Generalised anxiety disorder

31. Identify the false statement regarding anticholinergic drugs:

a) Orphenadrine has both antihistaminic and antimuscarinic actions.
b) Biperiden is the most M1 selective.
c) Benzhexol is the least M1 selective.
d) Procyclidine has a half-life of 36 hours.
e) Benzhexol may cause excitement.

32. Identify the antidepressant which has no active metabolite:

a) Venlafaxine
b) Fluvoxamine
c) Citalopram
d) Fluoxetine
e) Sertraline

33. The following are the serotonin receptor antagonists except:

a) Pindolol
b) Ketanserin
c) Yohimbine
d) Spiperone
e) Ondansetron

34. Identify the enzyme from the following which is not involved in the synthesis or in-activation of dopamine in a dopaminergic neurone:

a) Dopa-decarboxylase
b) Tyrosine hydroxylase
c) Monoamine oxidase
d) Dopamine β hydroxylase
e) Catechol-o-methyl transferase

35. The 'median effective dose' of a drug is the dose which shows therapeutic effect in:

a) 25% of patients
b) 60% of patients
c) 75% of patients
d) 50% of patients
e) 100% of patients

36. In depressive studies , the minimum percentage of decrease from baseline on a standard rating scale is:

a) 75%
b) 29%
c) 95%
d) 25%
e) 50%

37. Identify the incorrect statement regarding cytochrome P450 enzymes:

a) CYP1A2 - induced by smoking
b) CYP2C9 - induced by carbamazepine
c) CYP2D6 - inhibited by fluoxetine
d) CYP3A4 - inhibited by grapefruit juice
e) CYP2C19 - induced by fluvoxamine

38. Pharmacological actions of clozapine include the following except:

a) High affinity for cholinergic M_1 receptors
b) Low affinity for striatal D_2 receptors
c) D_2 partial agonism
d) Higher affinity for 5HT2A receptors than for striatal D_2 receptors
e) D_2 limbic selectivity

39. Identify the antianxiety drug which does not cause withdrawal syndrome on sudden discontinuation:

a) Lorazepam
b) Diazepam
c) Nitrazepam
d) Buspirone
e) Alprazolam

40. Identify the false statement from the following:

a) Morphine is a metabolite of codeine.
b) Naloxone is a pure competitive antagonist
c) Buprenorphine is a partial agonist at μ opiate receptor.
d) Acamprosate is an agonist at glutamate NMDA receptors.
e) Disulfiram inhibits aldehyde dehydrogenase.

41. Identify the false statement regarding drug interactions:

a) Diazepam displaces phenytoin from plasma proteins.
b) Carbamazepine decreases plasma concentration of risperidone.
c) Charcoal adsorbs tricyclic antidepressants.
d) Aspirin increases the risk of SSRI induced gastrointestinal bleeding.
e) Cimetidine reduces plasma tricyclic antidepressant levels.

42. One of the following drugs used in the treatment of general anxiety disorder, acts at alpha 2 delta subunit of calcium channel:

a) Buspirone
b) Diazepam
c) Sertraline
d) Pregabalin
e) Duloxetine

43. Inducers of CYP3A4 include the following except:

a) St John's wort
b) Phenytoin
c) Valproate
d) Rifampicin
e) Carbamazepine

44. Identify the drug from the following that can be used to treat tardive dyskinesia:

a) Bromocriptine
b) L-dopa
c) Orphenadine
d) Tetrabenazine
e) Amantadine

45. The following drugs cannot be used to treat obsessive compulsive disorder without comorbidity except:

a) Monoamine oxidase inhibitor
b) SNRI
c) Antipsychotic drug as monotherapy
d) Benzodiazepine
e) SSRI

46. Identify the false statement regarding lithium from the following:

a) Effective in acute mania.
b) Can reverse neutropenia.
c) Effective as an adjunct to antidepressant in treatment of depression
d) Has shown efficacy in reducing impulsivity
e) Abrupt lithium discontinuation does not lead to rebound mania.

47. Identify the least suitable SSRI in patients with narrow angle glaucoma and depression:

a) Paroxetine
b) Citalopram
c) Fluoxetine
d) Escitalopram
e) Fluvoxamine

48. Identify the false statement regarding clinical trials measuring the efficacy of a drug:

a) Pragmatic trials have more internal validity than external validity.
b) Randomisation increases the internal validity of a trial.
c) Crossover trials are useful in rare diseases.
d) Randomised clinical trials measure clinical efficacy of a drug in ideal conditions.
e) Pragmatic trials measure clinical effectiveness of a drug.

49. Identify the false statement from the following regarding the actions of drugs at the benzodiazepine receptor:

a) Full agonists are anxiolytics.
b) Partial agonists are mild anxiolytics.
c) Antagonists have no effect of their own.
d) Partial inverse agonists are anxiolytics.
e) Full inverse agonists are pro-convulsants.

50. The following are the inhibitors of uridine diphosphate glucuronosyl transferases except:

a) Diazepam
b) Clomipramine
c) Lorazepam
d) Carbamazepine
e) Valproic acid

1. Common side-effects of SSRIs include the following except:
Ans. b) Paraesthesia

2. Identify the false statement regarding antidepressant drugs:
Ans. d) Persistent adverse effects do not occur.

3. Peripheral antimuscarinic effects of the antipsychotic drugs include the following except:
Ans. e) Pyrexia

4. The antidopaminergic action of the AP drugs on the tuberoinfundibular pathway results in the following except:
Ans. c) Akathisia

5. Pharmacodynamic drug interactions include the following except:
Ans. a) Enzyme induction

6. Signs of lithium intoxication include the following except:
Ans. d) Lens opacity

7. Identify the false statement about plasma level determinations of the psychotropic drugs:
Ans. e) Useful if assessed after 5 doses.

8. Identify the false statement regarding risperidone long acting injection:
Ans. c) Therapeutic levels reach after one week after the first injection.

9. Risk of seizures is high with the following except:
Ans. a) Moclobemide

10. Depression is a recognised side effect of the following except:
Ans. e) Valproate

11. Risks of using SSRIs in pregnancy include the following except:
Ans. e) Increased neural tube defects

12. Lithium use in pregnancy is associated with the following in the neonate except:
Ans. e) Rash

13. Dosage reduction is recommended in hepatic impairment for the following except
Ans. a) Amisulpride

14. Which of the following is preferably avoided if glomerular filtration rate is <10ml/min:
Ans. d) Lithium

15. Zuclopenthixol acetate should not be used for the following except:
Ans. e) Patients who require repeated injections of short acting antipsychotic drugs.

16. Identify the false statement regarding caffeine:
Ans. d) Decreases clearance of lithium.

17. Drugs that can cause 'antabuse' reaction with alcohol include the following except:
Ans. e) Aspirin

18. Side-effects of reboxetine include the following except:
Ans. b) Blurred vision

19. Animal models used in testing the efficacy of antidepressants include the following except:
Ans. e) Pre pulse inhibition

20. Predictors of good response to lithium include the following except:
Ans. d) Rapid cycling bipolar illness

21. Action of sodium valproate include the following except:
Ans. a) Enhances GABA-transaminase

22. Lithium has shown efficacy in the following conditions except:
Ans. e) Adjunct to antidepressants in general anxiety disorder

23. Identify the false statement regarding benzodiazepines:
Ans. b) Inverse agonists at the BZD receptor enhance the action of GABA.

24. Placebo response is common in the following except:
Ans. d) Dementia

25. All but one of the following increase the risk of antidepressant induced hyponatraemia:
Ans. c) Obesity

26. Following antidepressant drugs are relatively safe in diabetes except:
Ans. c) MAOI

27. Identify the antidepressant which is contraindicated in recent MI:
Ans. d) Amitriptyline

28. Side effects due to muscarinic cholinergic blockade include the following except:
Ans. c) Weight gain

29. Identify the approximate 5HT2A: D2 affinity ratio of clozapine from the following:
Ans. c) 30: 1

30. Indications for treatment with antidepressant drugs include the following except:
Ans. d) Dissociative disorder

31. Identify the false statement regarding anticholinergic drugs:
Ans. d) Procyclidine has a half-life of 36 hours.

32. Identify the antidepressant which has no active metabolite:
Ans. b) Fluvoxamine

33. The following are the serotonin receptor antagonists except:
Ans. c) Yohimbine

34. Identify the enzyme from the following which is not involved in the synthesis or in-activation of dopamine in a dopaminergic neurone:
Ans. d) Dopamine β hydroxylase

35. The'median effective dose' of a drug is the dose which shows therapeutic effect in:
Ans. e) 100% of patients

36. In depressive studies , the minimum percentage of decrease from baseline on a standard rating scale is:
Ans. e) 50%

37. Identify the incorrect statement regarding cytochrome P450 enzymes:
Ans. e) CYP2C19 - induced by fluvoxamine

38. Pharmacological actions of clozapine include the following except:
Ans. c) D_2 partial agonism

39. Identify the antianxiety drug which does not cause withdrawal syndrome on sudden discontinuation:
Ans. d) Buspirone

40. Identify the false statement from the following:
Ans. d) Acamprosate is an agonist at glutamate NMDA receptors.

41. Identify the false statement regarding drug interactions:
Ans. e) Cimetidine reduces plasma tricyclic antidepressant levels.

42. One of the following drugs used in the treatment of general anxiety disorder, acts at alpha 2 delta subunit of calcium channel:
Ans. d) Pregabalin

43. Inducers of CYP3A4 include the following except:
Ans. c) Valproate

44. Identify the drug from the following that can be used to treat tardive dyskinesia:
Ans. d) Tetrabenazine

45. The following drugs cannot be used to treat obsessive compulsive disorder without comorbidity except:
Ans. e) SSRI

46. Identify the false statement regarding lithium from the following:
Ans. e) Abrupt lithium discontinuation does not lead to rebound mania.

47. Identify the least suitable SSRI in patients with narrow angle glaucoma and depression:
Ans. a) Paroxetine

48. Identify the false statement regarding clinical trials measuring the efficacy of a drug:
Ans. a) Pragmatic trials have more internal validity than external validity.

49. Identify the false statement from the following regarding the actions of drugs at the benzodiazepine receptor:
Ans. a) Full agonists are anxiolytics.

50. The following are the inhibitors of uridine diphosphate glucuronosyl transferases except:
Ans. d) Carbamazepine

Paper 52

1. Risk factors for side effects of antipsychotic drugs
   Link up to 4 risk factors (a – g) with each of the side effects of anti psychotic drugs (1 – 3) below:

   a) Male gender
   b) Advancing age
   c) Higher dosage
   d) Female gender
   e) High potency conventional anti psychotics
   f) Drug naïve patient
   g) Younger age

   1) Dystonia _____

   2) Parkinsonism _____

   3) Tardive dyskinesia _____

2. Animal models
   Match up to 3 of the animal models (a – f) used for drug research for each of the disorders (1–3) below:

   a) Prepulse inhibition
   b) Learned helplessness
   c) Tail suspension test
   d) Forced swim test
   e) Vogel test
   f) Elevated plus maze test

   1) Anxiety _____

   2) Schizophrenia _____

   3) Depression _____

3. Teratogenic defects
   Match up to 4 of teratogenic defects (a – g) with each of the drugs (1– 3) below:

   a) Spina bifida
   b) Cleft lip
   c) Coarctation of aorta
   d) Hypospadias
   e) Ebstein's anomaly
   f) Limb defects
   g) Macrosomia

   1) Lithium _____

   2) Carbamazepine _____

   3) Sodium valproate _____

4. Targets of action of antiepileptic drugs
   Match up to 6 of the anti epileptic drugs (a – h) with their targets of action (1– 2) below:

   a) **Pregabalin**
   b) **Carbamazepine**
   c) **Topiramate**
   d) **Valproate**
   e) **Gabapentin**
   f) **Lamotrigine**
   g) **Zonisamide**
   h) **Riluzole**

   1) **Voltage sensitive sodium channels** _____

   2) **Voltage sensitive calcium channels** _____

5. Rate limiting enzymes
   Match the synthesis of neurotransmitters (1 – 4) with their rate limiting enzyme(a – f) below.

   a) **Acetyl Cholinesterase**
   b) **Tyrosine hydroxylase**
   c) **Dopa decarboxylase**
   d) **Tryptophan hydroxylase**
   e) **Histidine decarboxylase**
   f) **Choline Acetyltransferase**

   1) **Synthesis of Serotonin** _____

   2) **Synthesis of Dopamine** _____

   3) **Synthesis of Noradrenaline** _____

   4) **Synthesis of Histamine** _____

6. Antidotes for drug overdoses
   Match each of the drugs (1 – 3) below with their correct antidotes in cases of their overdose (a – h) below:

   a) **Flumazenil**
   b) **Naltrexone**
   c) **Buprenorphine**
   d) **Methadone**
   e) **Disulfiram**
   f) **Physostigmine**
   g) **Apomorphine**
   h) **Naloxone**

   1) **Anticholinergic overdose** _____

   2) **Benzodiazepine overdose** _____

   3) **Heroin overdose** _____

7. Clinical trials

Link the types of clinical trial (a–f) with the appropriate description (1-4) below:

a) Pragmatic trial
b) Cluster trial
c) n-of-1 trial
d) Open trial
e) Controlled trial
f) Crossover trial

1) A single subject is blindly given two or more treatments in succession. _____

2) All patients in a particular location are randomized. _____

3) Interventions are directed at groups rather than individuals. _____

4) Patients receive different interventions by acting as their own controls. _____

8. Contraindications

Match each of the clinical scenarios (1 – 4) with one drug (a – g) which is contraindicated in that scenario:

a) Carbamazepine
b) Disulfiram
c) Thiazide diuretics
d) Antimuscarinic drugs
e) Amisulpride
f) Reboxetine
g) Clonidine

1) A 27 year old male with history of chronic treatment resistant schizophrenia but currently stable on clozapine.

_____

2) A 24 year old female with history of alcohol dependence currently presenting with binge drinking.

_____

3) A 33 year old male with history of schizophrenia, stable with antipsychotic treatment, has developed severe tardive dyskinesia.

_____

4) A 26 year old male on treatment with lithium for acute mania. _____

9. Co-transmitter peptides
   Link each of the neurotransmitters (1 – 3) with up to 3 co-transmitter peptides (a – i) below:

   a) Encephalin
   b) Cholecystokinin
   c) Somatostatin
   d) Neurotensin
   e) Substance P
   f) Thyrotrophin releasing hormone
   g) Vasoactive intestinal peptide
   h) Luteinizing hormone releasing hormone
   i) Motilin

   1) Dopamine _____

   2) Serotonin _____

   3) GABA _____

10. Mechanisms of action of antipsychotic drugs
    Link each atypical antipsychotic drug (1 – 3) with up to 2 mechanisms of action (a – h) below:

    a) Short dopamine 2 receptor off time
    b) Dopamine 3 receptor antagonism
    c) 5HT2A receptor antagonism and dopamine 2 receptor antagonism
    d) dopamine 2 receptor partial agonism
    e) Histamine receptor antagonism
    f) Multiple weak receptor affinities including dopamine 2
    g) 5HT3 antagonism
    h) Pure dopamine 2 receptor antagonism

    1) Quetiapine _____

    2) Risperidone _____

    3) Aripiprazole _____

11. Response to drug treatment
    Match up to three of statements (a – h) with each of the drug classes (1 – 3) below:

    a) Occurrence of discontinuation syndrome
    b) 33% respond and 67% fail to respond in depression
    c) 90% continue to respond and 10% relapse given initial response
    d) Monotherapy insufficient in 20% of patients
    e) 50% continue to respond and 50% relapse when this is given instead of treatment which
       produced an initial response
    f) Potential in bipolar maintenance
    g) 67% respond and 33% fail to respond in depression
    h) 10% of patients fail to achieve remission on this treatment

    1) All major classes of antidepressants _____

    2) Placebo _____

    3) Atypical antipsychotic drugs _____

12. Mechanisms of action

Match up to three of (a – h) with each of the mechanisms of action (1 – 3) below:

a) Acute dystonia
b) Urinary retention
c) Sedation
d) Blurred vision
e) Weight gain
f) Headache
g) Nausea
h) Bradykinesia

1) Dopamine 2 receptor antagonism _____

2) Histamine 1 receptor antagonism _____

3) Muscarinic receptor antagonism _____

13. Treatment

For each of the scenarios (1 – 3) state up to 3 of a-h which are not associated below:

a) Previous alcohol dependence
b) Inadequate early treatment
c) Dysthymia
d) Increased relapse rates
e) Functional impairment
f) Increased suicide risk
g) Refractoriness to psychological therapy
h) Continuing mild illness

1) Partial response in depression _____

2) Treatment resistant schizophrenia _____

3) Current alcohol dependence _____

14. Neurotransmitter functions

Match up to three of functions (a – i) with the neurotransmitter systems (1 – 3) below:

a) Mood
b) Working memory
c) Energy levels
d) Mirror neuron activation
e) Obsessive compulsive phenomena
f) Attention
g) Procedural memory
h) Lactation
i) Analgesia

1) Noradrenergic systems _____

2) Endogenous opiate systems _____

3) Serotonergic systems _____

15. Serotonergic systems
    Match up to two of (a – h) with each of the serotonergic systems (1 – 3) below:

    a) **Control of appetite and eating behaviour**
    b) **Insomnia**
    c) **Nausea and vomiting**
    d) **Sexual dysfunction**
    e) **Diarrhea**
    f) **Akathisia**
    g) **Anxiety**
    h) **Obsessive compulsive phenomena**

    1) **Serotonergic projections to the hypothalamus** _____

    2) **Serotonergic projections to the brainstem** _____

    3) **Serotonergic projections to the gut** _____

16. Pharmacokinetic parameters
    Match up to three options from (a – g) with each of the pharmacokinetic parameters (1 – 3) below:

    a) **Determines the maintenance dose**
    b) **Increases with lipid solubility**
    c) **Does not apply to drugs with zero order kinetics**
    d) **Determines the loading dose**
    e) **Increased by enzyme inducers**
    f) **Determines the dose interval**
    g) **Increases with the larger volume of distribution of the drug**

    1) **Clearance** _____

    2) **Volume of distribution** _____

    3) **Half-life** _____

Paper 52

1. Risk factors for side effects of antipsychotic drugs
   Link up to 4 risk factors (a – g) with each of the side effects of anti psychotic drugs (1 – 3) below:

   Ans. 1) a, e, f, g
   2) b, c, d, e
   3) b, d

2. Animal models
   Match up to 3 of the animal models (a – f) used for drug research for each of the disorders (1 – 3) below:

   Ans. 1) e, f
   2) a
   3) b, c, d

3. Teratogenic defects
   Match up to 4 of teratogenic defects (a – g) with each of the drugs (1 – 3) below:

   Ans. 1) e, g
   2) a
   3) a, c, d, f

4. Targets of action of antiepileptic drugs
   Match up to 6 of the anti epileptic drugs (a – h) with their targets of action (1 – 2) below:

   Ans. 1) b, c, d, f, g, h
   2) a, c, e, g, h

5. Rate limiting enzymes
   Match the synthesis of neurotransmitters (1 – 4) with their rate limiting enzyme(a – f) below.

   Ans. 1) d
   2) b
   3) b
   4) e

6. Antidotes for drug overdoses
   Match each of the drugs (1 – 3) below with their correct antidotes in cases of their overdose (a – h) below:

   Ans. 1) f
   2) a
   3) h

7. Clinical trials
   Link the types of clinical trial (a – f) with the appropriate description (1 – 4) below:

   Ans. 1) c
   2) a
   3) b
   4) f

8. Contraindications
   Match each of the clinical scenarios (1 – 4) with one drug (a – g) which is contraindicated in that scenario:

   Ans. 1) a
   2) b
   3) d
   4) c

9. Co-transmitter peptides
   Link each of the neurotransmitters (1 – 3) with up to 3 co-transmitter peptides (a – i) below:

   Ans. 1) a, b
   2) e, f, a
   3) c, i

10. **Mechanisms of action of antipsychotic drugs**

    Link each atypical antipsychotic drug (1 – 3) with up to 2 mechanisms of action (a – h) below:

    Ans. 1) a, f
         2) c
         3) d

11. **Response to drug treatment**

    Match up to three of statements (a – h) with each of the drug classes (1 – 3) below:

    Ans. 1) a, c, g
         2) b, e
         3) d, f

12. **Mechanisms of action**

    Match up to three of (a – h) with each of the mechanisms of action (1 – 3) below:

    Ans. 1) a, h
         2) c, e
         3) b, c, d

13. **Treatment**

    For each of the scenarios (1 – 3) state up to 3 of (a – h) which are not associated below:

    Ans. 1) a
         2) a, c, h
         3) h

14. **Neurotransmitter functions**

    Match up to three of functions (a – i) with the neurotransmitter systems (1 – 3) below:

    Ans. 1) a, c, f
         2) a, i
         3) a, e

15. **Serotonergic systems**

    Match up to two of (a – h) with each of the serotonergic systems (1 – 3) below:

    Ans. 1) a
         2) b, c
         3) e

16. **Pharmacokinetic parameters**

    Match up to three options from (a – g) with each of the pharmacokinetic parameters (1 – 3) below:

    Ans. 1) a, c, e
         2) b, d
         3) f, g

Bibliography

American Psychiatric Association. DSM-IV TR. Diagnostic and Statistical Manual of Mental Disorders. 4th ed. Washington DC: American Psychiatric Association; 2000.

Anderson IM, Reid IC. Fundamentals of Clinical Psychopharmacology. London & New York:Taylor & Francis Group; 2004

Baxter K. Stockley's Drug Interactions. 9th ed. London: Pharmaceutical Press; 2010

Bazire, S. Psychotropic Drug Directory. Aberdeen: Healthcomm UK Ltd; 2010

Begg EJ. Instant Clinical Pharmacology. Oxford: Wiley-Blackwell; 2002

Brunton LL, Lazo JS, Parker KL (eds). Goodman & Gilman's The Pharmacological Basis of Therapeutics. 12th ed. New York, NY: McGraw Hill; 2011

Chee HN, Keh-Ming L, Singh BS, Chiu EY. Ethno-psychopharmacology: Advances in Current Practice (Cambridge Medicine). Cambridge: Cambridge University Press; 2008

Cookson, J, Taylor,D, Katona C. Use of Drugs in Psychiatry. 5th ed. London: Gaskell; 2002

Davies DM, Ferner RE, de Glanville (eds). Davies's Textbook of Adverse Drug Reactions. London: Chapman and Hall Medical; 1999

Davis KL, Charney D, Coyle JT, Nemeroff C (eds). Neuropsychopharmacology. The Fifth Generation of Progress. Philadelphia: Lippincott Williams & Wilkins; 2002

Dhillon S, Kostrzewski A. Clinical Pharmacokinetics. London: Pharmaceutical Press; 2006

Fawcett J, Stein DJ, Jobson KO. Textbook of Treatment Algorithms in Psychopharmacology; New York: John Wiley & Sons; 1999

Gelder M, Andreason N, Lopez-Ibor J, Geddes J. New Oxford Textbook of Psychiatry. Vol 2. Oxford: Oxford University Press; 2009

Gorwood P, Hamon M. Psychopharmacogenetics. London: Springer; 2006

Green WH. Child and Adolescent Psychopharmacology. 4th ed. Philadelphia, PA: Lippincott Williams & Wilkins; 2007

Haddad P, et al. Adverse Syndromes and Psychiatric Drugs – A Clinical Guide. Oxford: OUP; 2005

Jacobson SA, Pies R, Katz IR. Clinical Manual of Geriatric Psychopharmacology. American Psychiatric Publishing; 2007

Joint Formulary Committee. British National Formulary (BNF) 62. 62nd ed. London: Pharmaceutical Press; 2011

Karalliedde K, Henry J (eds). Handbook of Drug Interactions. London: Arnold; 1998

Kruk ZL, Pycock CJ. Neurotransmitters and Drugs. 3rd ed. London: Chapman and Hall; 1991

Kalyna Z, Bezchlibnyk-Butler BJ, Jeffries J. Clinical Handbook of Psychotropic Drugs. 16th ed. Ashland, OH: Hogrefe; 2006

King DJ. Seminars in Clinical Psychiatry. Gaskell; 2004

Lee A. Adverse Drug Reactions. 2nd ed. London: Pharmaceutical Press; 2006

Leonard BE. Fundamentals of Psychopharmacology. 3rd ed. Chichester: Wiley; 2003

Lerer B. Pharmacogenetics of Psychotropic Drugs. New York: Cambridge University Press; 2002

Mrazek DA. Psychiatric Pharmacogenomics. New York: Oxford University Press; 2010

Musa MN (ed). Pharmacokinetics and Therapeutic Monitoring of Psychiatric Drugs. Springfield, Illinois: Charles C Thomas; 1993

Owens DGC. A Guide to the Extrapyramidal Side-effects of Antipsychotic drugs. Cambridge: Cambridge University Press; 1999

Pedro R. Ethnicity and Psychopharmacology (Review of Psychiatry, Vol 19, No. 4). Washington DC: American Psychiatric Press; 2000

Pies RW. Handbook of Essential Psychopharmacology. 2nd edn. New York: Oxford University Press; 2005

Puri BK, Tyre PJ. Sciences Basic to Psychiatry. Edinburgh: Churchill Livingstone; 1992

Rang HP, Dale MM, Ritter JM, Flower RJ. Rang and Dale's Pharmacology. 6th ed. Edinburgh: Churchill Livingstone Elsevier; 2007

Reveley MA, Deakin JFW (eds). The Psychopharmacology of Schizophrenia. London: Arnold Publishers; 2001

Sadock BJ, Sadock VA, Ruiz P. Comprehensive Textbook of Psychiatry, Vol. 2. 9th edn. Philadelphia, PA: Wolters Kluwer Health/Lippincott Williams & Wilkins; 2009

Schatzberg AF, Nemeroff CB (eds). Textbook of Psychopharmacology. 4th edn. Washington DC: American Psychiatric Publishing, Inc; 2009

Schatzberg AF, Cole JO, DeBattista C. Manual of Clinical Psychopharmacology. 7th edn. Washington DC: American Psychiatric Publishing Inc; 2010

Schwab M, Kaschka WP, Spina E. Pharmacogenomics in Psychiatry. Basel: Karger; 2010

Shiloh R, Stryjer R, Nutt D, Weizman A. Atlas of Psychiatric Pharmacotherapy. 2nd ed. London: Informa Healthcare; 2006

Sibley DR., Hanin I, Kuhar M, Skolnick P (eds). Handbook of Contemporary Neuropharmacology. 3 Vols. Hoboken, NJ: Wiley Interscience; 2007

Spiegel R. Psychopharmacology – An Introduction. 4th ed. Chichester: Wiley & Sons; 2003

Stahl SM. Antipsychotics and Mood Stabilizers: Stahl's Essential Psychopharmacology. 3rd edn. New York: Cambridge University Press; 2008

Stahl SM. Essential Psychopharmacology. Neuroscientifi c basis and Practical Applications. 3rd edn. Cambridge, UK: Cambridge University Press; 2008

Stahl SM. Essential Psychopharmacology: The Prescriber's Guide. Cambridge, UK: Cambridge University Press; 2009

Stein DJ, Lerer B, Stahl SM. Evidence-based Psychopharmacology; Cambridge University Press; 2005

Taylor D, Paton C. Case Studies in Psychopharmacology. 2nd edn. London: Martin Dunitz; 2002

Taylor D, Paton C, Kapur S. The Maudsley Prescribing Guidelines. 10th edn. London: Informa Healthcare; 2009

Tyrer P. Psychopharmacology of Anxiety. Oxford: Oxford University Press; 1989

Walsh BT (ed). Child Psychopharmacology. Washington DC: American Psychiatric Association; 1998

Weber WW. Pharmacogenetics. 2nd edn. Oxford University Press; 2008

World Health Organization. The ICD-10 Classification of Mental and Behavioural Disorders; 1992. WHO website. www.who.int/entity/classifications/icd/en/GRNBOOK.pdf. Accessed 13 Oct 2011.

Wright P. Core Psychopharmacology. In: Wright P, Phelan M, Stern J, eds. Core Psychiatry. 2nd edn. London: Elsevier Saunders; 2006